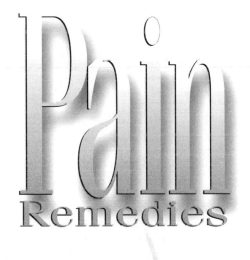

Pain
Remedies

Over 1,000
Quick&Easy

Pain

Remedies
From Little Ouches to Big Aches

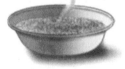

By Philip Goldberg
and the Editors of *PREVENTION* Magazine

Medical Adviser: Willibald Nagler, M.D., Physiatrist-in-Chief,
New York Hospital–Cornell Medical Center and Professor of
Rehabilitation Medicine, Cornell University Medical College, New York City

RODALE PRESS, INC.
EMMAUS, PENNSYLVANIA

Copyright © 1997 by Philip Goldberg

Library of Congress Cataloging-in-Publication Data

Goldberg, Philip, 1944–
    Over 1,000 quick and easy pain remedies from little ouches to big aches /
by Philip Goldberg and the editors of Prevention Magazine.
        p.   cm.
    Includes index.
    ISBN 0–87596–285–8 hardcover
    1. Pain—Popular works. 2. Analgesia—Popular works.
I. Prevention Magazine. II. Title: Over one thousand quick and easy pain remedies from little ouches to big aches.
RB127.G65   1997
616'.0472—DC21   97–8239

Distributed in the book trade by St. Martin's Press

2 4 6 8 10 9 7 5 3 1 hardcover

Editorial Staff for *Pain Remedies*

Senior Managing Editor: Edward Claflin
Editors: Susan G. Berg, Julia VanTine
Contributing Editor: Jared T. Kieling
Assistant Research Manager: Anita C. Small
Editorial Researcher: Paris Muchanic
Copy Editors: Kathryn A. Cressman, Marybeth McFarland, Karen Neely
Associate Art Director: Faith Hague
Cover and Book Designer: Vic Mazurkiewicz
Technical Artist: Eugenie Delancy
Manufacturing Coordinator: Patrick T. Smith
Office Manager: Roberta Mulliner
Office Staff: Julie Kehs, Bernadette Sauerwine

Rodale Health and Fitness Books

Vice President and Editorial Director: Debora T. Yost
Executive Editor: Neil Wertheimer
Design and Production Director: Michael Ward
Research Manager: Ann Gossy Yermish
Copy Manager: Lisa D. Andruscavage
Studio Manager: Stefano Carbini
Book Manufacturing Director: Helen Clogston

Contents

Foreword ix

◆◆◆

Angina 1

Ankle Pain 4

Arthritis 7

Back Pain 11

Bedsores 17

Blisters 20

Breast Pain 23

Broken Nails 28

Bunions 30

Burns 33

Bursitis 36

Calf Pain 39

Cancer Pain 43

Canker Sores 48

Carpal Tunnel
Syndrome 51

Chafing 54

Childbirth Pain 57

Cold Sores 60

Corneal Burns
and Abrasions 63

Corns 66

Cuts and Scrapes 69

Denture Pain 72

Diverticulosis 75

Ear Pain 78

Endometriosis 83

Eye Pain 87

Eyestrain 91

Facial Pain 95

Fissures and Abscesses 98

Foot Pain 101

Gallbladder Pain 105

Gas Pain 108

Genital Herpes 111

Gout 114

Gum Pain 117

Hangover 123

Headache 126

Heartburn 131

Heel Pain 134

Hemorrhoids 138

Hip Pain 141

Ingrown Toenail 146

Intercourse Pain 150

Irritable Bowel
Syndrome 154

Kidney Stones 157

Knee Pain 161

Menstrual Pain 166

Migraine 170

Muscle Cramps 176

Muscle Spasms 181

Neck Pain 185

Penile Pain 190

Phantom Limb Pain 193

Pizza Burn 197

Postoperative Pain 199

Razor Burn 203

Repetitive Strain
Injury 206

Sciatica 210

Shingles 215

Shinsplints 219

Shoulder Pain 223

Side Stitches 227

Sinus Pain 230

Sore Throat 234

Splinters 239

Stomach Pain 242

Stubbed Toe 248

Sunburn 251

Temporomandibular
Disorder (TMD) 255

Tennis Elbow 261

Testicular Pain 265

Tongue Pain 268

Toothache 273

Ulcers 278

Varicose Veins 282

Windburn 286

Wrist Pain 289

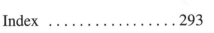

Index 293

Foreword

Why is it crucial to have a book that focuses solely on pain remedies? Because pain is the central element in most patient-physician interactions. Studies have shown that pain accounts for the majority of calls or visits to primary care physicians, who constitute about 70 percent of all practicing physicians.

We live in a time when costs for health services are increasing, financial coverage by HMOs is shrinking, and individual medical savings accounts are gaining increased attention from the experts. These developments mean, more and more, that responsibility for one's health care is being shifted to the individual. As a result, self-help advice and self-help literature have become increasingly important.

For these reasons, *Pain Remedies* is a much-needed, timely addition to the self-help medical library. If you are experiencing pain and want to know what to do about it, just identify what part of your body hurts and turn to that entry in the book. You'll quickly find a selection of practical, effective self-care strategies. You'll also find guidelines to let you know when you should see your doctor. Thanks to the information provided in this book, you will be quite knowledgeable about your condition—which will make it much easier for your doctor to prescribe treatment.

What makes this book so unique is that the self-help advice comes from specialists, who have expertise about the specific body systems in which pain can originate. For example, a physiatrist—who specializes in physical medicine and rehabilitation—offers suggestions for relieving musculoskeletal pain, or pain in the muscles, bones, and joints. A gastroenterologist answers your questions about digestive discomfort. A dentist provides tips for dealing with toothache and mouth pain.

Most of these specialists are associated with large academic medical centers. These institutions are famous for being on the cutting edge of new developments in the treatment and prevention of pain. You'll find out how you can make these medical breakthroughs work for you—starting now.

Some of the remedies in the following pages contain elements that might be considered "alternative" rather than "traditional" medicine. The fact is, a so-called alternative solution has often served as the basis for what would later be considered a traditional, or more scientific, approach.

For example, aspirin—one of the most widely prescribed pain medications—has been known to us since the seventeenth century. Back then, it was "prescribed" for joint pain and was taken either orally, as a bitter-tasting extract made from the bark of a willow tree, or topically, by applying it right on the affected joint. Later, when its chemical constituents were better understood, it became available in tablet form. But it wasn't until 1972 that John Vane, a Nobel Laureate, linked the pain-relieving action of aspirin to its ability to block inflammation-producing prostaglandins. These days, other nonsteroidal anti-inflammatory drugs (NSAIDs), such as ibuprofen and naproxen, work on the same physiological principle as aspirin. Yet no one would think of aspirin as an alternative therapy anymore.

Likewise, it used to be considered "bad medicine" to recommend therapeutic exercises for the treatment of pain in the lumbar, or lower back, area. Doctors favored the surgical approach, because it seemed logical to attempt to alter the anatomical structures that were thought to be causing pain. Now, however, it is widely recognized and accepted that therapeutic exercises play a major role in the treatment of lower back pain. When you do these exercises, your muscles adapt to bone changes that take place over time, and the nagging pain generally subsides. Here again, what was once thought to be alternative medicine is not alternative anymore.

Often we know through observation and experience that certain remedies work—but we can't explain how they work. Nor can we "prove" them until we make certain advances in scientific exploration and techniques. For centuries, humans have been applying ice to aching body parts, but no one really understood how that would relieve pain. Through research, we now know that ice decreases pain sensations by lowering the temperatures of sensory nerves. This minimizes their ability to conduct signals from the area that hurts to the nerve centers that register pain.

In recent years, we've witnessed an explosion in medical knowledge and in the development of sophisticated, high-tech tools for disease diagnosis and treatment. Still, the fact remains that large numbers of people continue to suffer from pain. And those numbers will continue to grow: Thanks to progress in the medical sciences, we're now living longer—which means we have more years and more opportunities to experience injuries and health problems. The day may come when we know how to reduce all kinds of pain to tolerable levels without the powerful side effects that we now see with certain strong medications.

In the meantime, there are many things you can do for yourself—some of them surprisingly simple. The more you know about taking care of your own aches and pains, the better off you will be.

Even when you do need professional medical care, you can make a big difference in the healing process by becoming actively involved in your treatment. Personally, I do not believe that a doctor should take a position of absolute authority in his relationship with a patient. Instead, the two of you should develop a cooperative partnership, deciding together what needs to be done to bring about your return to good health. The information provided in this book should help to enhance the quality of interaction and discussion between you and your doctor.

Pain Remedies is a treasure chest of sound, essential advice on the subject of pain management. No matter where you hurt, you'll find a tip or two that can help you feel better fast. Keep this book handy— and use it in good health.

Willibald Nagler, M.D.
Physiatrist-in-chief, New York Hospital–Cornell
Medical Center and professor of rehabilitation
medicine, Cornell University
Medical College, New York City

Angina

A common symptom of heart disease, angina occurs when some part of the heart does not receive enough blood because the vessels that feed it—called the coronary arteries—are blocked. In other words, your heart isn't getting the oxygen it needs. Commonly, you will feel a squeezing sensation in the center of your chest, perhaps radiating to your shoulder, up your neck, and down your arm.

Angina pain might recede once you rest. But most likely, it will return: Your coronary arteries are blocked, and you run a greater risk of having a heart attack. This risk is no less if you happen to be female. "Women are just as much at risk of developing angina and atherosclerosis," says Richard A. Helfant, M.D., clinical professor of medicine and director of cardiology training at the University of California, Irvine, and author of *Women Take Heart.* "Women need to take angina symptoms seriously, especially after menopause."

Get to the Root of the Pain

Angina pain can be minimized. But the key is to remedy the condition's underlying cause—heart disease—as well as the symptoms. The following heart-smart advice from experts can help you treat both cause and symptoms and help alleviate the pain.

Rest. If you experience an angina attack, sit or lie down immediately, says Dr. Helfant.

Take your medicine. If you've experienced angina in the past, your doctor has most likely advised you to take nitroglycerin the instant you have an attack. But this drug can also be taken before angina occurs.

"Take your nitroglycerin before doing anything that tends to produce the symptoms," says Charles K. Francis, M.D., chairman of the department of medicine at Harlem Hospital Center in New York. "If you know that your angina bothers you when you mow the lawn, for example, take your nitroglycerin before you head outside."

Take no more than three nitroglycerin tablets, says Dr. Helfant. If you continue to experience pain after 15 to 30 minutes, despite having taken nitroglycerin, "call for an ambulance or have someone take you to the emergency room," he says.

Preventing a Heart Attack

The best defense against angina pain is to prevent future attacks, say experts. That means taking steps to prevent your coronary arteries from closing any further. Here is what the experts suggest.

Take a daily dose of aspirin. If you have angina, take one baby aspirin a day or half a regular aspirin every other day, recommends Dr. Helfant. "Aspirin has been shown to be of clear-cut value in preventing heart attacks," he says. "It makes the platelets circulating in the blood less likely to clump together and form a clot."

Kick the cancer sticks. Smoking constricts the coronary arteries, says Dr. Helfant—just what you don't need with angina pain.

Send your cholesterol south. According to National Cholesterol Education Program (NCEP) guidelines, total cholesterol should be below 200 milligrams per deciliter (mg/dl), "bad" low-density lipoprotein (LDL) cholesterol should be below 130 mg/dl, and "good" high-density lipoprotein (HDL) cholesterol should be above 35 mg/dl. The best way to help lower cholesterol naturally is to avoid high-fat, high-cholesterol foods, says Dr. Francis.

When you eat is as important as what you eat, says John Zamarra, M.D., a cardiologist and assistant clinical professor of medicine at the University of California, Irvine. "Eat your main meal of the day at lunch and have a light meal in the evening," he says. "Your body can't digest fat as efficiently at night as it can during the day."

When to See the Doctor

Report any attack of angina pain to your doctor, says Charles K. Francis, M.D., chairman of the department of medicine at Harlem Hospital Medical Center in New York.

You should also consult a doctor if your angina symptoms increase in frequency, severity, or duration, says Richard A. Helfant, M.D., clinical professor of medicine and director of cardiology training at the University of California, Irvine, and author of *Women Take Heart*. "Chest pain due to coronary disease may not be the crushing, terrible pain you might expect," he notes.

If you are experiencing chest pain but have not been diagnosed with angina, get medical help immediately if your pain lasts for more than a minute or occurs with any of the following symptoms: shortness of breath; dizziness; radiation of the pain to the neck, jaw, shoulders, or arms; sweating; or nausea.

Get your blood moving. "Regular exercise can help reduce stress, control your weight, reduce your blood pressure, and increase your level of 'good' HDL cholesterol," says Dr. Helfant. Taking a brisk walk for ½ hour a day, four times a week is all it takes. Consult your doctor before beginning a walking regimen or other fitness routine, he adds.

Reduce your pressure. High blood pressure is a primary culprit in heart disease, says Dr. Francis. "If you have angina, your doctor will monitor your blood pressure to reduce the likelihood that it will lead to future problems," he says.

Try to stay tranquil. Try to manage stress as best you can, perhaps by learning a relaxation technique such as meditation, says Dr. Zamarra. And find a bit of serenity whenever and wherever you can: "Be kind to yourself and never underestimate the power of a loving spouse and faith in something bigger than yourself," he says. "Happiness that comes from within is healing."

Ankle Pain

You did it again—stumbled on the steps of the escalator at the mall. Teenagers snickered. Pain and humiliation fought for your attention. Humiliation won.

Now, the morning after your mishap, the humiliation has faded, but the pain in your ankle hasn't. You park yourself on the sofa, weighing whether to hobble to work or stay home and catch the early-morning movie.

Essentially a hinge, the ankle is the meeting place of three bones and a system of ligaments, tendons, and muscles. We put so much wear and tear on our ankles that they are prone to injury, especially sprains and strains. A sprain involves damage to the ligaments, while a strain pertains to the muscle and tendons.

And if you think a sprained ankle is most likely to be a runner's problem, guess again. Sedentary folks who slip, stumble, or otherwise take a misstep may be more likely to sprain an ankle than athletic types.

Prompt treatment will speed healing and reduce the risk of further injury, say experts. "Twenty percent of sprains lead to chronic ankle pain," says Carol Frey, M.D., a foot and ankle surgeon at the Orthopedic Hospital in Los Angeles. "Lots of people say, 'It's just a sprain,' and don't get treatment. Then the ligaments heal poorly, or scar tissue forms between the bones at the joint."

When You Trip Up

A sore ankle is impossible to ignore. But doctors have found some low-pain ways to get you up and walking again. Try these tips the next time you trip over your own two feet.

When to See the Doctor

If your ankle is so swollen that you can't put on your shoe or put weight on your leg, get medical attention, says Enyi Okereke, M.D., chief of foot and ankle surgery at the University of Pennsylvania Medical Center in Philadelphia.

"You may have a severe sprain with torn ligaments or even a fracture," says Dr. Okereke. "Many times people walk around with a fracture, thinking it's just a sprain." Either condition can cause major problems.

Serve up some RICE. We're not advocating that you appeal to Uncle Ben. RICE stands for rest, ice, compression, and elevation. Here's how it works, explains Dr. Frey.
- Rest your ankle for the first day or two.
- Ice your ankle, three to four times daily, but no longer than 20 minutes at a time. (And always have a towel between the ice or ice pack and your skin so that you don't get frostbite.)
- Compress the injury by wrapping it with an elastic bandage.
- Elevate your ankle above the level of your heart.

RICE will limit bleeding in the joint and swelling in the tissues, thereby easing the pain.

Soothe with heat. After two to three days, apply warm compresses, says Arthur H. Brownstein, M.D., a physician in Princeville, Hawaii, and clinical instructor of medicine at the University of Hawaii School of Medicine in Manoa. Here's his unusual remedy.
- Boil fresh grated gingerroot, then let it cool a little.
- Make a compress by soaking a washcloth in the warm brew.
- Place the compress over the injured ankle.

According to Dr. Brownstein, ginger draws out toxins and hastens healing.

Take some tablets of relief. If your ankle really hurts, consider easing the pain with an over-the-counter nonsteroidal anti-inflammatory drug (NSAID) such as ibuprofen, suggests Dr. Frey. Follow the directions on the product label.

But don't ignore lingering pain or try to cover it up with over-the-counter painkillers, says Phillip A. Bauman, M.D., clinical instructor in orthopedic surgery at the Columbia University College of Physicians and Surgeons and associate attending physician of orthopedic surgery at St. Luke's/Roosevelt Hospital Center, both in New York City. You need to be aware of pain to keep from reinjuring vulnerable muscles or tendons, he says.

Building a Stronger Ankle

Once you have sprained your ankle, you have to be extra careful, say experts. "If you don't strengthen your ankle after you sprain it, you're likely to injure it again in the future," says Dr. Bauman.

"After the pain and swelling in your ankle subsides, it's important to strengthen the ligaments, tendons, and muscles," agrees Dr. Frey. She recommends the following exercise, developed by William S. Case, president of Case Physical Therapy in Houston.

- Sit on the floor with your legs straight out in front of you.
- Wrap a towel around the ball of the foot on the same side as your injured ankle and grip the ends of the towel in your hands.
- Pull the towel toward you, flexing your foot with it. Hold for 10 seconds and relax.
- Then point your toes forward into the towel, using your arms for resistance. Hold for 5 seconds.
- Repeat 10 times.

Arthritis

Anyone who thinks arthritis affects only little old ladies who wear bifocals and sensible shoes, raise your hand—if you can. Can't lift your hand without flinching? You have lots of company. About 40 million of us have some form of arthritis, and the pain of this condition can range from occasional twinges to bona fide aches. More women develop the condition than men.

Arthritis means joint inflammation. It is an umbrella term for more than 100 different disorders. Generally speaking, there are two kinds of arthritis: osteoarthritis and rheumatoid arthritis, says Cody Wasner, M.D., a rheumatologist and clinical assistant professor at Oregon Health Sciences University in Eugene. Osteoarthritis, the type that most people get, causes pain, swelling, and limited movement in joints and connective tissue. Rheumatoid arthritis, a more serious form of the disease, is caused by a breakdown in the body's immune system.

There's no cure for arthritis—at least not yet. The good news is that there's a lot you can do to alleviate the pain and stiffness and keep the creakiest of joints moving. Try these strategies from the experts.

Give arthritis the cold treatment. Wrap an ice pack in a towel and apply it to the painful joint for no longer than 20 minutes at a time, says Dr. Wasner. If you don't have an ice pack, he adds, use a bag of frozen peas. Remove the ice for 10 to 20 minutes between applications.

Blanket sore muscles with heat. While heat should not be applied to inflamed joints, it can soothe achy muscles and overall stiffness, says Dr. Wasner.

Apply heat (in the form of a hot-water bottle) for 15 to 20 minutes every 2 to 3 hours, recommends Eric P. Gall, M.D., chairman of the department of medicine at Finch University of Health Sciences/

When to See the Doctor

If your arthritis pain is mild, "it's fine to mention it to your doctor the next time you see him," says Eric P. Gall, M.D., chairman of the department of medicine at Finch University of Health Sciences/Chicago Medical School. But see a doctor immediately if the pain doesn't subside within a week, especially if it is accompanied by fever or weakness.

Chicago Medical School. "Moist heat is especially soothing first thing in the morning if you're stiff," he adds.

Try to stay active. Regular exercise can help keep your joints flexible and your muscles strong, say experts. Try working out in a warm pool, if possible; the buoyancy of the water reduces the impact on your joints. Check your local Y for an Arthritis Foundation/ YMCA aquatic program. Or ask your doctor to recommend an exercise routine that's right for you.

Limber up with yoga. Tight, tense muscles can cause wear and tear on the joints, says Arthur H. Brownstein, M.D., a physician in Princeville, Hawaii, and clinical instructor of medicine at the University of Hawaii School of Medicine in Manoa. A gentle regimen of yoga can help keep your muscles supple and flexible. If you're just getting started, consult a physical therapist or massage therapist who has been trained in yoga, he advises. Or look in the Yellow Pages under "Yoga Instruction."

Flex, flex, flex. Put a painful joint through its full range of motion two or three times a day, recommends Dr. Gall. Flex the joint as far as you can in one direction, then in the other. "When you feel discomfort, try to move the joint farther," he says. "If you feel pain, stop."

Anoint the ache with ointment. Rub aching joints with an arthritis ointment that contains capsaicin, the ingredient that gives chili peppers their heat, suggests Dr. Wasner. "There's evidence that capsaicin is helpful."

You might also try Tiger Balm, a traditional Chinese salve sold in health food stores, says Dr. Brownstein. "Rub it on the affected area before you go to sleep."

Take a wax dip. If your hands or feet hurt, try a paraffin dip, suggests Dr. Wasner. "Buy a paraffin bath at a medical supply store," he says. "This device heats the wax and keeps it at a therapeutic temperature. The wax adheres to your skin and stays warm for some time. When the wax cools, you peel it off and return it to the container for reuse."

Prevent the Pain before It Strikes

Not only can you relieve arthritis pain, you can take steps to prevent it in the first place. Here's how.

Watch your weight. Carrying extra pounds puts extra stress on your joints. In fact, some research has suggested a link between being overweight and developing arthritis in the knee.

Try to stay tranquil. Stress and fatigue can make arthritis pain worse, says Dr. Wasner. "Stress-busting activities such as meditation, yoga, guided imagery, and prayer can be helpful for some people," he says.

Eat fish. There's some evidence that fish rich in omega-3 fatty acids, such as herring, mackerel, salmon and tuna, may help reduce arthritis pain, says Melvyn Werbach, M.D., a physician in Los Angeles who specializes in nutritional medicine and the author of *Healing with Food.* Some people prefer to take fish oil supplements (available in drugstores or health food stores).

Cut back on fat. What you *don't* eat—in this case, dietary fat—may also ease your joints. "Dietary fat, especially saturated fat, appears to have an adverse effect on rheumatoid arthritis," says Dr. Werbach.

Pain Relief for Every Part

Here are some pain-relief tips that target the body parts most affected by arthritis: feet, knees, hands, and shoulders.

For your toes. If your toes overlap, insert a spacer between them. If the pain is located in the joint where the toe meets the foot, try a metatarsal bar, suggests Frederick McDuffie, M.D., director of Piedmont Hospital Arthritis Center in Atlanta. You'll find both of these devices in drugstores and medical supply stores.

For your feet. Fill one basin with cool water and another with warm water. Soak your feet for 5 minutes in the cool water, then 5 minutes in the warm water. Continue until the warm water cools.

For your knees. Use a hydrocollator—a pad filled with silicon gel that you heat up in a microwave, suggests Dr. McDuffie. These are also available in drugstores and medical supply stores.

Or sit in a bath that's as warm as you can stand it. "Make sure that you have grab bars to help you get in and out of the tub," he says.

For your hands and wrists. Dip a hand towel in a basin of water, then wring it out, rotating your wrists as you do. This exercise will work your hands, fingers, wrists, and forearms, experts say.

If your hands are swollen, wear tight-fitting gloves (such as Isotoner) whenever you can, "including to bed," says Dr. McDuffie.

"The joint at the base of the thumb is commonly affected by arthritis," says Edward A. Rankin, M.D., chief of orthopedic surgery at Providence Hospital in Washington, D.C. "Look for a special splint, called a gamekeeper splint, which you fasten around the thumb and wrist."

For your shoulders. "Get into the shower and let water that's comfortably hot run over the painful shoulder," says Dr. McDuffie. "Then reach out to the side, keeping your shoulder relaxed, and climb your hand up the shower wall with your fingers. Climb as high as you can, rest for 5 seconds, and try to go a bit higher. Then slowly walk your fingers back down."

Back Pain

You bent down, picked up the laundry basket, straightened up, and . . . *yeeow!* Pain cut through your back like a sword. What happened? You have lifted heavier loads than this hundreds of times before.

Doesn't matter. Back pain will seize any opportunity to strike—while you're hefting a sack of groceries, slouching in front of the TV, hunching over your desk, standing in line for movie tickets, even sleeping the wrong way. And once it hits, back pain can be relentless.

It starts in different ways with different people. You might feel a mild twinge when you sit, walk, drive, tie your shoes, or turn to answer the phone. Or—if you're less fortunate—you'll feel as though you have been stabbed in the back with an ice pick. Back pain is also an equal-opportunity affliction: Four of every five of us will have back pain at some point in our lives, says Garth Russell, M.D., clinical professor of orthopedics at the University of Missouri—Columbia School of Medicine and senior surgeon at Columbia Spine Center, both in Columbia.

Speedy Relief for an Aching Back

Most back pain is caused by muscle spasms—abnormal contractions that squeeze the blood vessels in some area of the back, depriving that tissue and muscle of nourishment. The good news is that most back pain responds to self-care. Even better news: If managed properly, most back pain resolves itself within two weeks.

These tips can help you manage your pain.

Turn the pain on "cold." "Ice is especially helpful when the pain is most acute—the first two to three days," says Richard Aptaker,

Pick It Up Right

The easiest way to hurt your back is to pick up something the wrong way. But what is the right way? Here is the advice of Richard Aptaker, D.O., chief of the department of physical medicine and director of the Spine Clinic at Kaiser Permanente Medical Center in San Francisco.

- Stand close to the object that you want to lift, with your feet shoulder-width apart.
- Bend at the knees (not the waist), keeping your back straight or bent slightly forward.
- Lift with your thigh muscles, not with your arms. (Just think of your arms as hooks that grab the load.)

Be sure that you don't twist your body while you're lifting. "Once you're upright, point your toes in the direction that you want to move and pivot with your legs and feet," says Garth Russell, M.D., clinical professor of orthopedics at the University of Missouri—Columbia School of Medicine and senior surgeon at the Columbia Spine Center, both in Columbia. That way you'll turn your whole body instead of twisting your back. Always keep the object close to your body.

To lift a bulging suitcase, says Dr. Russell, "Stand beside it, bend at the knees, grasp the handle, and straighten up."

D.O., chief of the department of physical medicine and director of the Spine Clinic at Kaiser Permanente Medical Center in San Francisco. "It helps reduce inflammation and relaxes the muscle spasm. Apply ice to the painful area for about 15 minutes at a time every 2 hours, six to eight times a day."

But don't put ice directly on your skin, advises Thomas Rizzo, Jr., M.D., a physiatrist in the department of physical medicine and rehabilitation at the Mayo Clinic in Jacksonville, Florida. "It could cause frostbite," he says. "Put a thin towel between the ice and your skin."

Heat it up—maybe. Not all experts advise heat. "I recommend using ice when back pain is caused by overuse or spasm, and heat if the discomfort is related to stiffness of the joints or muscles," says Dr. Rizzo. "Heat loosens the muscles and makes them more flexible."

And if you're using heat, put your hot-water bottle or heating pad on your back, rather than lying directly on it, says Thomas B. Curtis, M.D., a physiatrist at the Virginia Mason Medical Center in Seattle. "You don't want to fall asleep and burn yourself."

Wear a corset. "Muscles support the bones, disks, and nerves that make up the spine," says Dr. Rizzo "Weak muscles put more pressure on those structures. So wearing a soft, elasticized corset can help support the back."

But don't depend on a corset for too long, he adds. "Prolonged use of a corset can make the muscles weaker."

Get into position to heal. When your back hurts, trying the following positions may make you more comfortable, says Dr. Aptaker. Lie on your back on the floor with a pillow or rolled-up towel under your knees and another under your neck. Then raise your arms over your head to give your spine a bit of a stretch.

Or you can lie on your side with one pillow between your knees and another under your head, says Dr. Aptaker. You might also place a rolled-up towel under your waist.

Sit right. Sitting can aggravate back pain, according to Dr. Aptaker. "It's one of the worst things that you can do," he says. If you have to sit, "use a chair with good back support and armrests, which reduce pressure on your back. Also, put a pillow behind your lower back and keep your feet flat on the floor with your knees bent."

Consider a pain reliever. Most experts recommend an over-the-counter nonsteroidal anti-inflammatory drug (NSAID) for back pain. "Take two 200-milligram tablets of ibuprofen, no more than three times a day," says Dr. Aptaker. While an NSAID can relieve pain quickly, "healing the inflammation can take 10 to 14 days," he notes.

When to See the Doctor

Not all back pain responds to self-treatment. "See a doctor if the pain is persistent, associated with a fever, or if you have weakness, numbness, or shooting pain in the leg," says Thomas B. Curtis, M.D., a physiatrist at the Virginia Mason Medical Center in Seattle. "This could be a sign of nerve damage."

If you have a chronic back problem, see your doctor if you notice a marked change in your usual symptoms, advises Richard Aptaker, D.O., chief of the department of physical medicine and director of the Spine Clinic at Kaiser Permanente Medical Center in San Francisco. "Also see a doctor if your pain is out of proportion to anything that you've experienced before, especially if it is associated with abdominal or stomach pain, chest pain, nausea, fever, chills, or loss of bladder or bowel control," he says.

Exercise the Pain Away

A strong back is a pain-free back, and most experts recommend back exercises. "It's important for the muscles of the back and abdomen to be strong so that the spine is maintained in the proper position," says Dr. Rizzo. He recommends the following back exercises, designed to strengthen key muscles.

Note: If you're in severe pain, consult your doctor before attempting these exercises, and stop immediately if the pain gets worse.

- Lie flat on your back with your legs stretched out in front of you. Pull one knee toward your chest with both hands, placing them on your thigh behind and above your knee until you feel a stretch—but not pain—in your back. Hold for about 30 seconds. Rest a few seconds, then repeat with the other knee.
- Lie on your back with your knees bent and your feet flat on the floor. Using your stomach muscles, suck in your belly while tilting your hips upward until your lower back is flat against the floor. Hold for 10 seconds. Relax 1 to 2 seconds, then repeat 10 times.

- Lie on your back with your knees bent, your feet on the floor, and your arms folded across your chest. Press your lower back to the floor. Then lift your head slowly until your shoulders are off the ground. Hold for 10 seconds. Lower yourself back to the floor. Repeat 10 times.
- Kneel on all fours, keeping your back parallel to the floor. Arch your back upward like a cat. Hold for 2 seconds. Lower your back to the original position. Repeat 5 to 10 times.
- Lie facedown on the floor with a pillow or two under your hips and stomach. While keeping your hips on the pillows, raise your left arm and right leg simultaneously, until the muscles of your lower back and buttocks feel tight. Hold for 2 seconds. Lower your arm and leg. Repeat with the right arm and left leg. Do 10 sets.

Staying Active Can Help, Too

While you should avoid doing anything that aggravates your back pain, "it's important to get active as soon as possible," says Dr. Curtis. "Continued bed rest can cause your muscles to atrophy or tighten and encourage the psychological perception of disability. Too much rest can also delay the use of therapies that are more likely to be more helpful."

And it only takes a couple days of rest to get ready to go again. "Studies show that a day or two of rest is as effective as seven or more," adds Dr. Aptaker.

Here are some simple ways to stay active.

Take a hike. Walking is the most convenient—and possibly most effective—exercise for the back, says Dr. Aptaker. He recommends taking a 20-minute walk three to five times a week.

Plunge into the pool. Swimming is the ideal exercise if you have a back problem, says Dr. Russell. "In a pool you're buoyant," he says. "The water supports you. Your muscles can move freely without a lot of resistance, so you don't put stress on your back."

Try tai chi. Unlike other types of martial arts, the ancient Chinese practice of tai chi is gentle. And that means it's perfect for a painful back, says Stella Shigenaka, a physical therapist at the Institute of Progressive Physical Therapy in Los Angeles. "I recommend it to back patients because it increases their body awareness, involves every part of the body, and can be done by anyone of any age," she says.

Stretch Out with Yoga

Yoga can help stretch the back muscles, says Mary Pullig Schatz, M.D., a pathologist and yoga instructor in Nashville and author of *Back Care Basics*. "Yoga can help strengthen the back while you're also learning the principles of correct movement," she says. But don't overdo these exercises, cautions Dr. Schatz; you could hurt your back.

Dr. Schatz suggests working with a yoga teacher who has treated people with back injuries. She also recommends the following exercises.

- Kneel on all fours with your knees directly under your hips and your hands directly under your shoulders. Don't raise your head. Without arching your back, raise one arm and stretch it forward. Hold for a few breaths, then lower your arm. Repeat on the other side.
- Kneeling on all fours, straighten one leg, then raise it. Don't over-arch your lower back. Hold for several breaths, then lower your leg. If lifting your leg hurts your back, keep your knee bent and lift it only a few inches off the floor. Repeat on the other side.
- Stand about a foot away from a wall, with your feet 6 to 8 inches apart. Place your hands (with fingers pointing up) on the wall at shoulder height and shoulder-width apart. Pushing your hands into the wall, step back as you bend forward from your hips (not your waist). If that's painful, step toward the wall and position your hands a little higher until you feel a comfortable stretch in the muscles in the backs of your legs. Don't overarch or round your back. Hold the pose for one to three breaths.

Bedsores

Bedsores aren't a pleasant topic. But they can be a fact of life for anyone who can't care for themselves, from an ailing parent confined to a wheelchair to a bedridden friend facing an extended recuperation from an accident or chronic condition.

Also called pressure ulcers, bedsores are caused by constant pressure on one part of the body, usually on areas that cover a bony area, such as the lower back, hips, buttocks, and heels. Under this unrelenting pressure, tissue is starved of oxygen and nutrients.

While bedsores are usually the unwelcome bedfellows of more serious health concerns, they're no trivial matter. "The biggest complication of bedsores is infection," says Bruce Ferrell, M.D., assistant professor of medicine and geriatrics at the University of California, Los Angeles, UCLA School of Medicine. "The infection can spread throughout the skin, bone, or even the bloodstream, which can be extremely serious."

Sore No More

The good news is that there is no reason to suffer. The pain of bedsores can be relieved, and—with proper care—even prevented, says Diane Krasner, R.N., a nurse consultant in Baltimore who specializes in chronic wound care. Here are some suggestions from Krasner and other experts.

Put sores under cover. Keep bedsores covered to prevent infection, says Krasner. "Moist dressings tend to be less painful," she says.

And since bedsores tend to hurt most when the dressings are changed, Dr. Ferrell suggests taking a pain reliever (such as acetaminophen) beforehand.

When to See the Doctor

If you're at risk for bedsores, you're most likely under a doctor's care already. But tell your doctor or nurse about any sign of ulceration, say experts. "If you notice a reddened area that doesn't go away, get a doctor's help as quickly as possible," says Diane Krasner, R.N., a nurse consultant in Baltimore who specializes in chronic wound care.

Don't assume that if a bedsore doesn't hurt, it's not serious, adds Krasner. Constant pressure tends to numb the skin, and other conditions such as paralysis or diabetes may reduce the ability to feel pain.

Ask about OTCs. If your bedsores hurt continuously, says Dr. Ferrell, you may want to ask your doctor about taking over-the-counter medication at regular intervals, not just when the pain flares. Acetaminophen, aspirin, or another pain reliever may be appropriate. But be sure to consult your doctor before taking these medications regularly.

Try zinc and vitamin C. While some research suggests that these nutrients help speed wound healing, studies are inconclusive, says Dr. Ferrell. If you want to try supplementation, discuss the idea with your doctor first, he advises. In the meantime, do eat a well-balanced diet, which ensures that you're getting your daily allowance of vitamin C and zinc.

Keep moving. Since bedsores are caused by constant pressure, "move around as much as you can," says Dr. Ferrell. "If you're in a wheelchair, try to change your position at least once an hour. If you're in bed, try to turn at least once every 2 hours." If you can't move by yourself, ask your nurse or partner to help.

Use de-pressurizing devices. Special beds, mattresses, seat cushions, and other devices can help ease the discomfort of bedsores, says Krasner. Ask your doctor which of these products might be right for you.

Stay dry. "Keep your skin clean and dry," says Krasner. "People who sweat heavily or who are incontinent are more likely to develop pressure ulcers." But don't go overboard: Having excessively dry skin can lead to sores, too. "If you have dry skin, use a moisturizer after you bathe," says Dr. Ferrell.

Use the power of your mind. Some people with pressure ulcers have found stress-relieving techniques such as imagery, meditation, or prayer helpful in relieving the pain, according to Krasner.

Blisters

Couldn't resist that fancy pair of shoes, even though they rubbed the balls of your feet raw? Took a 2-hour hike in brand-new hiking boots? Raked an autumn's worth of leaves when you seldom grip anything wider than a pen? Chances are, the unrelenting friction between shoe or rake and skin caused the top two layers of skin to separate and the space between them to fill with fluid. That's what a blister is.

Most people get blisters on their feet, courtesy of ill-fitting shoes. But these little balloons of pain can sprout anywhere skin meets friction, especially on the hands and fingers. Here is how to deal with blisters and how to keep from getting them in the first place.

How to Pop a Blister

Once you have a blister, the best way to ease the pain is to pop it, says Glenn Gastwirth, D.P.M., deputy executive director of the American Podiatric Medical Association. But you have to do it right. Start by sterilizing a needle or pin under a flame, allowing it to cool to room temperature before using it. Then swab the blister with alcohol and— holding the needle parallel to your skin—pierce the edge of the blister.

You'll need to pierce more than once, says Rodney Basler, M.D., a dermatologist in private practice in Lincoln, Nebraska. "Puncture the blister three times in the first 24 hours—once immediately, then every 12 hours," he says.

After you pierce the blister, swab it with an antiseptic and cover it with a bandage to protect it from dust and dirt, says Dr. Gastwirth. If the blister is on your foot, "don't make the bandage so thick that it becomes a new source of irritation," he advises.

When to See the Doctor

In most cases you can soothe a blister's sting on your own. But consult a doctor if you see signs of infection such as pus, swelling, or redness, says Rodney Basler, M.D., a dermatologist in private practice in Lincoln, Nebraska.

Beware the Cruel Shoes

No matter how stylish they are, tight shoes are a ticket to Blister City. But too-loose shoes can set your dogs barking, too: "Even a small amount of friction can form a blister," says Dr. Gastwirth. Here's how to keep your feet blister-free.

Wear shoes that fit. The toe box of your shoes should be high enough for you to easily wiggle your toes, while the heel of the shoe should neither slide nor pinch, says Dr. Gastwirth.

Break in shoes gradually. While new shoes should feel comfortable the minute you leave the store, many people find that they need to break them in. "Don't wear new shoes longer than 2 hours the first day," says Dr. Gastwirth.

Lubricate hot spots. If you're prone to blisters in a particular area—say, your heel or the ball of your foot—slather the spot with petroleum jelly or a thick ointment, advises Joseph Ellis, D.P.M., a podiatrist in Ocean Side, California, and co-author of *Running Injury-Free.* "The lubrication will reduce the friction," he says.

Patch up problems. You might also wear a moleskin patch on these vulnerable areas, adds Dr. Gastwirth. Don't use adhesive bandages, however. "They slip and slide and cause the very friction that you're trying to avoid," he says.

Keep your dogs dry. Dust your feet liberally with foot powder, says Dr. Basler. Sweaty feet are blister-prone feet.

Search your sole. Wear inner soles to protect the balls of your feet, recommends Dr. Ellis. For instance, "Spenco makes an inner sole that provides a good cushion and reduces friction," he says. You will find inner soles in the foot-care section of drugstores or in sporting goods stores.

Inspect your shoes and socks. If you tend to develop blisters in the same spot, check your shoes for points of friction. "See if your shoe is excessively worn or if it has a torn seam or lining," suggests Dr. Gastwirth. Check your socks or stockings, too: A tear in a seam can cause friction, as can wadded-up hose.

Get your feet examined. If tight shoes or wayward hose aren't causing your blisters, consider consulting a foot specialist. High or fallen arches can cause blisters, says Allen Selner, D.P.M., a podiatrist at the Medstar Foot and Ankle Center in Studio City, California. So can a Charlie Chaplin gait—walking with your feet turned outward. To help correct the foot problem and prevent future blisters, a podiatrist may prescribe orthotics, corrective devices that fit in your shoes.

Breast Pain

The first thing you should know about breast pain is that fewer than 5 percent of the women who see a doctor for this condition have breast cancer. The second thing you need to know is that you should see a doctor to rule out breast cancer anyway.

About half of all women experience breast pain (mastalgia) at some time in their lives, according to Mary Ann Braun, a registered nurse and coordinator of the Comprehensive Breast Center at the Georgetown University Medical Center in Washington, D.C. But even when your breasts have gotten the all clear from your doctor, you may still have to contend with garden-variety breast pain, caused by everything from your normal menstrual cycle—a phenomenon known as cyclical breast pain—to cysts and infections. Two-thirds of women experience cyclical pain.

Fortunately, you can ease ordinary achy breasts with everything from vitamins and herbs to massage and simple changes in your diet and habits. These tips can help keep your breasts virtually pain-free.

The Nutrition Link

What you put in your mouth can help ease breast pain or aggravate it, according to some doctors. So eat to heal with these expert-recommended strategies.

Get your E. Consider taking 400 international units of vitamin E per day, says Sherry Goldman, a nurse practitioner at the UCLA Breast Center in Los Angeles. "If you don't get relief, try 800 international units," she says.

Making It through Your Mammogram

Some women experience discomfort during a mammogram. "If your breasts are already tender, a mammogram can exacerbate your discomfort," says Gillian Newstead, M.D., medical director of breast imaging at New York University Medical Center in New York City. If your breast pain is related to your menstrual cycle, schedule a mammogram for just after your period, when your breasts are least tender.

And try to schedule your mammogram with an experienced technician: She can significantly reduce the discomfort you may feel, says Dr. Newstead.

But if getting a mammogram hurts, consider taking an over-the-counter pain medication before you undergo this proce-dure, suggests William Dooley, M.D., director of the Johns Hop-kins Breast Center in Baltimore.

You should notice some benefit within four to six weeks of starting the supplement, says William Dooley, M.D., director of the Johns Hopkins Breast Center in Baltimore.

Note: Experts suggest that you consult your doctor before taking more than 600 international units of vitamin E per day.

Be generous with Bs. Taking 300 to 500 milligrams of vit-amin B_6 a day may help prevent breast pain, says Norman Schulman, M.D., an obstetrician/gynecologist at Cedars–Sinai Medical Center in Los Angeles.

That's because vitamin B_6 is a natural diuretic—that is, it helps release water from the body, says Cynthia M. Watson, M.D. a family practitioner in private practice in Santa Monica, California. If you opt to try B_6 for breast pain, make sure to get the Daily Value of the rest of the Bs, either in a multivitamin or a B-complex supple-ment, she says.

Note: You should talk to your doctor before taking more than

100 milligrams of vitamin B_6 a day, since high levels of B_6 can cause uncoordination while walking and numbness in the feet.

Cut back on fat. A diet of chips and cheeseburgers may satisfy your taste buds, but your breasts may bear the brunt of a fat-laden diet. Conversely, reducing your fat intake can help ease achy breasts. "When women had severe breast pain related to their menstrual cycles, and they reduced their intake of dietary fat to 15 percent of their caloric intake, their breasts were less tender, swollen, and lumpy," says Melvyn Werbach, M.D., a physician in Los Angeles who specializes in nutritional medicine and the author of *Healing with Food.* Don't eliminate fat from your diet entirely, however; your body needs it to absorb vitamin E.

Avoid caffeine. That means coffee, tea, cola, and—alas—chocolate. And don't think that you can cheat by drinking decaf: "Even decaffeinated coffee contains some caffeine," says Dr. Dooley.

Hide your saltshaker. Cut back on salt, advises Dr. Schulman. Cyclical breast pain is associated with fluid retention. Reducing your sodium intake is particularly important a week or so before your period, he says.

More Pain-Away Strategies

Once you have adjusted your diet, there is still more that you can do to relieve breast pain. Try these tips.

Massage your breasts. Daily massage can help ease breast pain by increasing the circulation to your breasts, says Felice Dunas, Ph.D., a licensed acupuncturist and a doctor of clinical Chinese medicine in private practice in Topanga, California. Here's how to do it. Place your hands on your breasts with your fingers spread and your nipples in your palms. Squeeze and release your fingers as you massage the circumference of your breasts.

Wear a bra to bed. A well-fitting bra can help lessen non-cyclical breast pain, says Braun. She recommends wearing a support

---

When to See the Doctor

If breast pain is not related to your menstrual cycle, or if you have pain and you're over age 50, see a doctor, experts advise. "Also, see your doctor if the pain is persistent and is located in one particular area of your breast," says Gillian Newstead, M.D., medical director of breast imaging at New York University Medical Center in New York City.

Other conditions that warrant a trip to the doctor include nipple discharge, associated shoulder pain, and, of course, a lump, says Norman Schulman, M.D., an obstetrician/gynecologist at Cedars/Sinai Medical Center in Los Angeles.

"Most painful lumps are not cancer," says William Dooley, M.D., director of the Johns Hopkins Breast Center in Baltimore. "But have any lump checked out by a doctor."

---

bra at night. "Running bras work well," she says. But use common sense when choosing a bedtime bra. "You're looking for support, not sex appeal," she says.

Learn to manage stress. "Stress can intensify breast pain by making you more sensitive to normal hormonal changes," says Braun. "So try to reduce the stress in your life, whether it's by listening to music or by learning a relaxation technique such as biofeedback."

Kick butts. "We don't know why, but smoking seems to be related to breast pain and the formation of small cysts," says Braun.

Try evening primrose oil. According to Braun, "Studies show that cyclical breast pain is substantially reduced or eliminated by taking evening primrose oil daily for three months." She suggests giving evening primrose oil (which is available in health food stores) a 90-day trial. "Follow the manufacturer's instructions for the lowest possible dosage. If it doesn't ease your breast pain within three months, it probably won't help," she says.

Note: Evening primrose oil may lead to miscarriage in some women, says Goldman. So don't take it if you're pregnant or if you want to be. Evening primrose oil can also cause diarrhea in some people.

Try non-Rx relief. An over-the-counter nonsteroidal anti-inflammatory drug (NSAID) such as ibuprofen can help ease breast pain, says Dr. Dooley.

But be aware that some over-the-counter medications, including some products for menstrual pain, contain caffeine or caffeine-like substances, says Braun.

Hormones Can Help, Too

Some women find that regulating their menstrual cycles with oral contraceptives helps reduce breast pain, says Gillian Newstead, M.D., medical director of breast imaging at New York University Medical Center in New York City. You'll need to discuss this option with your physician, of course.

Also, if you're postmenopausal and taking estrogen, you may experience breast pain several years after you begin hormone replacement therapy, says Dr. Dooley. He suggests asking your doctor to evaluate your dose.

Broken Nails

We use them as makeshift screwdrivers or pliers. We drown them in dishwater and coat them with chemicals. No wonder our nails so easily break.

Everything from a dry climate to constant immersion in hot water can cause nails to peel, split, and crack. And the pain can be considerable, especially if the nail splits to the quick.

If It's Broke, Fix It

The following tips can soothe the throb of a broken nail and help prevent painful splits in the first place.

Clip broken nails quickly. If you break a nail, cut it as short as you can, says C. Ralph Daniel, M.D., a dermatologist and clinical professor of dermatology at the University of Mississippi Medical Center in Jackson. This will keep the break from extending farther down your nail.

Bandage the break . . . maybe. If your nail is torn and raw, "apply an antibiotic ointment to help prevent infection, then cover the nail with a bandage," says Paul Kechijian, M.D., clinical associate professor of dermatology at the New York University School of Medicine in New York City and a dermatologist in Great Neck, New York.

No need to bandage a less-serious split, says Dr. Daniel. "A bandage will hold in heat and moisture, which can be detrimental."

Clip nails correctly. Cut your nails straight across, advises Dr. Daniel. Rounding the edges can cause an ingrown nail.

Don gloves. When you're doing household chores, wear heavy cotton gloves for dry work (such as gardening) and vinyl gloves

When to See the Doctor

A nail that's broken seldom requires medical attention. But a nail that's injured—by a slamming car door, for example—can be serious. You should see your doctor if you develop symptoms of infection, such as swelling, a fever, or the formation of pus, or if your nail is extremely painful. "If there's a lot of swelling or pain, you could have a broken bone, not just a broken nail," says C. Ralph Daniel, M.D., a dermatologist and clinical professor of dermatology at the University of Mississippi Medical Center in Jackson.

Also consult a doctor if you see blood under your nail, says Dr. Daniel. "Go to the emergency room within an hour to release the pressure beneath the nail," he says. "If the pressure is not released, it can damage the nail root." But don't be alarmed if your nail turns black, he adds. "It probably looks worse than it is."

with cotton gloves underneath for wet work (such as washing dishes), advises Dr. Daniel. "Your hands will sweat under the vinyl, and the cotton gloves will absorb the sweat," he explains.

Use an ocean of lotion. Massage your nails with plain petroleum jelly or a hand cream that contains 10 percent urea, recommends Dr. Kechijian. "Trapping moisture within the nails will help make them less brittle," he says.

Ration the nail polish remover. Touch up chipped polish instead of removing it completely, says Dr. Kechijian. The reason? Nail polish remover contains strong solvents that can make nails bone-dry, leaving them vulnerable to splits and cracks.

Try biotin. In animal studies, the vitamin biotin (available at drugstores and health food stores) has been shown to strengthen nails, says Dr. Kechijian. He recommends taking 2.5 milligrams of biotin a day. But don't expect overnight improvement: "It may take six months to see results," he says.

Bunions

Hallux valgus. It may sound like the name of a villain in a sci-fi flick, but it's actually the medical term for a bunion. And if you have one, the Darth Vader-ish moniker is fitting.

What's probably not fitting: your shoes. "Ninety percent of people who have bunions are women," says Carol Frey, M.D., a foot and ankle surgeon at the Orthopedic Hospital in Los Angeles. "And the most common cause of bunions is tight-fitting shoes, especially high heels."

A bunion is a misaligned joint that creates a bony prominence on the inside of the foot at the base of the big toe. This prominence forces the bone of the big toe to jut outward, jamming it at an angle toward the other toes. The resulting friction can cause swelling and inflammation of the bursa, a fluid-filled sac that cushions the joint, says Allen Selner, D.P.M., a podiatrist at Medstar Foot and Ankle Center in Studio City, California.

Soothing a Bunion's Sting

While the only way to correct the underlying misalignment is surgery, there are ways to ease bunion pain on your own, say foot experts. Here is what they suggest.

Put your bunions on ice. To help reduce the swelling and inflammation, apply ice to a painful bunion three or four times a day for 15 to 30 minutes at a time, says Rock Positano, D.P.M., co-director of the Foot and Ankle Orthopedic Institute at the Hospital for Special Surgery in New York City.

Shield your bunion. Bunion shields—little doughnut-shaped foam or felt pads that fit over a bunion—can ease the pressure caused

When to See the Doctor

Many people with bunions can relieve the pain on their own, say foot experts. But under certain circumstances, it's wise to have a doctor examine a bunion, says Allen Selner, D.P.M., a podiatrist at the Medstar Foot and Ankle Center in Studio City, California. "Consult a doctor if your bunion is extremely painful, if your big toe is hitting or hiding under your second toe, or if you can't bend your big toe," he recommends.

Also see a doctor if your bunion is paired with a callus on the inside of your big toe or on the ball of your foot, says Dr. Selner. A callus indicates that your body weight is not being properly transferred to your other joints, a condition that can be remedied with orthotics.

by your shoe, thereby lessening the pain, says Dr. Frey. You'll find bunion shields in drugstores or orthopedic supply stores.

S-t-r-e-t-c-h your shoes. Consider having a cobbler stretch your shoes over the bunion area, says Dr. Frey. "This can help ease painful pressure."

Step into comfortable footwear. Wear shoes with a rounded toe box, advises Dr. Frey. "Stick to glove leather or suede, which stretch, and avoid patent leather and synthetics, which don't 'give' as well."

Ditch the spikes. Choose heels that are less than 2¼ inches high and wear them no longer than 2 to 3 hours at a time, advises Dr. Frey. "If you can, kick off your heels when you're at your desk," she says.

Don sandals—or nothing. "Sandals won't put pressure on a bunion, so wear them whenever you can," says Dr. Frey. "Or go barefoot as often as you can, as long as it isn't dangerous."

Opt for orthotics. Orthotics are custom-fitted shoe inserts that redistribute your weight, thereby taking pressure off your bunion.

While you can buy ready-made orthotics in a drugstore, Dr. Frey recommends having a podiatrist or orthopedist fit you for the custom-made kinds.

Support your arches. Arch supports can't remedy bunion pain as effectively as orthotics, but they can be helpful, says Dr. Selner. "Spenco makes a very good arch support," he says. "Wearing them as often as possible may help the pain dramatically."

Splint a wayward toe. If your big toe is deformed and is causing pain, try wearing a splint (available at orthopedic supply stores), says Dr. Frey. "There are two kinds of splints: day splints, which you can wear in your shoes, and night splints, which you wear to bed."

Break out the NSAIDs. When your bunion swells and causes pain, consider taking an over-the-counter nonsteroidal anti-inflammatory drug (NSAID) such as ibuprofen, says Dr. Frey. "Take as directed on the package."

The Treatment of Last Resort

When it comes to banishing a bunion, having surgery should come last on your list of options, says Dr. Positano. "Try conservative treatment first," he advises. He will consider surgery if a bunion is extremely painful, if there is evidence of arthritis in the joint, or if the joint is deformed and is interfering with the functioning of the foot.

Experts agree on one thing: Don't have surgery for cosmetic reasons. "People often want surgery because they don't like the way their feet look or because they want to wear stylish shoes," says Dr. Positano. "It's not worth it. Surgery could make the problem worse."

Burns

Scalding tap water, the business end of a red-hot iron, a welt from a hot oven rack—all can cause an excruciatingly painful burn. So the most effective burn "remedy" is to avoid getting burned in the first place, says Libby Bradshaw, D.O., assistant professor of family medicine and community health at Tufts University School of Medicine in Boston.

Wise advice. But if you do get scalded or singed—and you probably will at some point—it's important to act fast, both to ease the pain and to save your skin. "What you do in the first few moments is crucial," says Karl N. Stein, M.D., staff surgeon at the Sherman Oaks Hospital Burn Center in Sherman Oaks, California.

Speedy Relief for Everyday Scorches

Common household burns are the kind that you get if you grasp the handle of a smoking saucepan or brush your calf against a blistering-hot radiator. They are known as first- or second-degree burns—resulting in redness, pain, and some blistering. More serious burns need a doctor's attention. But if you have just a common household burn, here are some tips to help squelch the pain.

Cool the burn. Flush the burn with cold water until the pain stops—as long as 20 to 30 minutes, says Dr. Stein. The heat from a burn continues to penetrate your skin even after you have removed the source of the heat, he explains. Cool water can help prevent the burn from going deeper.

If using running water is too painful, try a cold-water compress, suggests Joseph A. Witkowski, M.D., clinical professor of dermatology at the University of Pennsylvania School of Medicine in Philadelphia.

When to See the Doctor

Whether you should consult a doctor depends on the size and location of your burn, says Karl N. Stein, M.D., staff surgeon at the Sherman Oaks Hospital Burn Center in Sherman Oaks, California.

If the burn is small and not in a vulnerable area—the thigh or buttock, for example—you can treat it yourself, says Dr. Stein. But get to a doctor if you have even a small burn on your face, neck, armpit, or groin; if the burn is blistered and more than 2 inches in diameter; or if there is loss of feeling in the burned area.

Save the salve. Wait a while before applying any kind of salve or ointment to your burn, says Dr. Stein. "You have to neutralize the heat first," he says. "Otherwise, all the salve will do is baste the burn by keeping the heat inside."

When can you use salve? "Hours later," answers Dr. Stein. "If the burn is still painful and you develop a small blister, you can apply ointment to keep the burn lubricated."

Dr. Bradshaw recommends using an ointment containing the antibiotic bacitracin.

Aid with aloe. Use the cooling gel of the aloe vera plant to ease the pain of a superficial burn, says Dr. Stein. As with salves and ointments, you should hold off on the aloe to give the burn a chance to neutralize. At that point, he says, you can apply the gel twice a day, either directly from the leaf of the plant or in bottled form. "Use the clear kind, not the stuff with added coloring," he adds.

Keep the burn covered. Cover a burn with loose gauze, not an adhesive bandage, says Dr. Stein.

Or try an over-the-counter product called Spenco Second Skin. It's a thin layer of synthetic material that can be applied over superficial burns. "It's very soothing," says Dr. Witkowski. "Put one on your burn, and chill its replacement in the refrigerator." Why the fridge?

"Keeping the product cold makes it more effective as a pain reliever," he explains.

A bonus benefit to bandaging your burn: "A bandage reminds you that the burn is there, so you're less likely to bump it," says Dr. Bradshaw.

Speed healing with C. While it won't help reduce the pain, taking 500 to 1,000 milligrams of vitamin C a day can help heal a burn, according to Cynthia M. Watson, M.D., a family practitioner in private practice in Santa Monica, California.

Dr. Watson also suggests taking the mineral zinc. "Take 25 to 50 milligrams of zinc a day after you burn yourself and continue until the burn heals," she suggests.

Note: High levels of zinc can be toxic and should be taken only under the guidance of your physician.

Treating a Chemical Burn

Substances such as bleach, swimming pool acids, and various cleansers can burn your skin as readily as a heat source. But chemical burns require different treatment.

First and foremost, if you're burned by a chemical, follow the first-aid instructions on the product label. If you can't read the label, use common sense: "Wash off the substance immediately," says Dr. Stein. "If the chemical is in powder form, brush it off immediately, then wash your skin. If the chemical is on your clothes, remove them."

After you flood the burn with water, neutralize the chemical, says Dr. Stein. "If the burn was caused by an alkaline—like lye—neutralize it with something acidic, like vinegar," he says. If the burn was caused by an acid, irrigate the burn with an alkaline-based substance such as sodium bicarbonate or a liquid antacid. Then flood the burn with water once again.

Bursitis

Reaching for canned goods on high shelves in the supermarket didn't always make you wince. But now, raising your arm to retrieve a can of beans or box of pasta is an exercise in pain, and you're considering trading in shopping carts for take-out menus.

Think your aching shoulder may be signaling the first twinges of arthritis? Think again: You may have bursitis.

Bursitis is different from arthritis, although people often confuse the two because the pain can be so similar. In bursitis, the fluid-filled sacs that cushion the joints (bursae) become inflamed, most commonly from overuse. (In arthritis, it's the joints that become inflamed.) "The usual symptoms of bursitis are redness, swelling, and tenderness," says Ben W. Kibler, M.D., medical director of the Lexington Clinic Sports Medicine Center in Lexington, Kentucky. Only the doctor can tell you for sure whether you have bursitis or arthritis. But if you have had it before, you will recognize a flare-up again because of the pain.

Bursitis attacks the shoulder more often than any other part of the body, courtesy of a lifetime of playing golf or tennis, raking leaves, and washing the car. The shoulder bursa just wears out, much like an old fan belt. Chronic bursitis in the shoulder can develop into frozen shoulder, a condition in which the shoulder becomes virtually immobile. Bursitis can also flare up in the knee, hip, and elbow.

Shrug Off Bursitis Pain

The next time your bursitis acts up, fight back. Here's how to prevent the pain from getting the best of you.

Try ice. Wrap an ice pack in a towel and apply it to your sore shoulder or knee up to 20 minutes at a time, up to three times a day, says David Altchek, M.D., assistant professor of orthopedic surgery at Cornell University Medical College in New York City and team physician for the New York Mets. You might use an elastic bandage to keep the pack in place.

Avoid heat. Don't apply heat for the first two days, since it will aggravate the swelling, according to Dr. Kibler. After that, however, you may want to use a warm compress or a heating pad set on "low" to ease the pain.

Ease the ache with Arnica. After you ice the affected area, rub on some Arnica, suggests Cynthia M. Watson, M.D., a family practitioner in private practice in Santa Monica, California. This homeopathic remedy, which you apply directly to your skin, is used to reduce swelling and muscle soreness. You will find Arnica in health food stores or wherever homeopathic remedies are sold.

Massage away the pain. Gently massage the sore area to loosen the tissue, recommends Dr. Kibler. Be careful not to press too hard or too deep.

Take aspirin. Reduce the pain and swelling with an over-the-counter nonsteroidal anti-inflammatory drug (NSAID) such as aspirin, recommends Leon Robb, M.D., director of the Robb Pain Management Group in Los Angeles. Avoid aspirin and other NSAIDs, however, if you have gastrointestinal problems or a bleeding condition.

Work That Shoulder

While you should avoid activities that will put undue strain on your shoulder during a flare-up of bursitis, it's crucial to keep that shoulder supple, says Phillip A. Bauman, M.D., clinical instructor in orthopedic surgery at the Columbia University College of Physicians and Surgeons and associate attending physician of orthopedic surgery at St. Luke's/Roosevelt Hospital Center, both in New York City. A bursitis-ridden shoulder is much like a door hinge, he explains: "With neglect, the joint gets rusty and creaky." These gentle range-of-motion

When to See the Doctor

If your bursitis pain doesn't respond to self-treatment within two days, consult a doctor, says Ben W. Kibler, M.D., medical director of the Lexington Clinic Sports Medicine Center in Lexington, Kentucky. Severe pain also warrants a trip to the doctor: "Bursitis can be confused with other conditions, especially if the pain is located in your shoulder," he explains. "You could have rotator cuff tendinitis or a chip fracture."

exercises from experts can help build your shoulder's strength and preserve its flexibility.

• Put three 1-pound cans into a plastic bag. Stand at a counter and bend at the waist, placing your good arm on the countertop and cradling your head in the crook of that arm. Holding the bag of cans with your other hand, dangle your painful arm toward the floor and slowly move your arm in a circle. This exercise will pull your arm from beneath the bursa, says Dr. Robb. "Doing this regularly will help prevent the bursitis from getting worse," he says.

• Standing upright, bend your arm at the elbow so that the forearm of your painful arm is parallel to the floor. Hold a pillow against a wall and press the fist of your sore arm into it, suggests Dr. Altchek.

Then change your position so that your back is against the wall. Press the elbow of your sore arm back against the pillow, as if pushing someone who is standing behind you.

Finally, stand sideways to the wall. With your forearm still parallel to the floor, push the forearm against the pillow. Do each exercise 10 times and hold each position for 5 seconds. Perform the series five times a day.

• Raise your arms above your head, and then sway them from side to side, 10 to 15 times a day, advises Dr. Bauman. "This exercise can help maintain your range of motion and help prevent frozen shoulder." If you feel some discomfort, keep stretching. But if it hurts, stop and see a doctor.

Calf Pain

You're playing tennis. You hit a backhand and set yourself for the volley. It's a lob. You take off, lunging to reach the shot and . . . all of a sudden you hear a snap, and you can't move forward. You feel as though you have lost control of your left calf.

That's the scenario of a ruptured tendon. But calf pain isn't always so drastic. Often, it is a dull ache that grates your lower leg.

Sore calves can be triggered by foot problems—such as high arches or flat feet—or by ill-fitting shoes. Or the pain may be the result of a muscle tear, a partial rupture of the Achilles tendon, or the tendon inflammation called tendinitis.

There are also more serious medical conditions that can cause calf pain, such as phlebitis and intermittent claudication. The former refers to inflammation of a vein, while the latter means that arteries have become narrowed, resulting in an insufficient blood supply.

Problems like that will need to be treated by a doctor, of course. But if you have injured your calf or, more commonly, simply suffer from aching legs, you can get relief on your own.

Relief for Bleating Calves

Calf pain doesn't have to cramp your style. The tips below can stop the ache fast—and keep it from coming back.

RICE to the occasion. RICE means rest, ice, compression, and elevation. Rest an injured calf for the first day or two, ice the area for no more than 20 minutes at a time every 2 to 3 hours as needed, compress the leg with an elastic bandage, and elevate the leg above the level of your heart, if possible.

You can apply moist heat (such as a hot-water bottle) to the

When to See the Doctor

If your calf pain doesn't subside within a couple of days, see your doctor, says Myles J. Schneider, D.P.M., a podiatrist in Annandale, Virginia, and co-author of *The Athlete's Health Care Book.*

Also, consult a doctor immediately if walking a few blocks causes excruciating calf pain that stops when you sit. The pain could be caused by something minor, like fallen arches. But it could also be a symptom of either phlebitis or intermittent claudication, says John Cianca, M.D., assistant professor of physical medicine and rehabilitation at Baylor College of Medicine in Houston. These are both serious conditions that affect your circulation.

Phlebitis is an inflammation of a vein in the leg, says Dr. Schneider. "Usually, the painful area is warm and red," he says. Intermittent claudication, which feels much like a muscle cramp, is a sign that the arteries in your leg are partially blocked. Both can be relieved with treatment before they get worse, but a doctor should take care of them as soon as possible.

injury after the first 72 hours, says Allen Selner, D.P.M., a podiatrist at the Medstar Foot and Ankle Center in Studio City, California. "Moist heat is more effective than dry heat," he says.

Rub and wrap. Once the swelling recedes, rub your injured calf with a pain-relieving balm (such as BenGay) and wrap it in a plastic wrap, says Dr. Selner. Then top that wrap with an elastic bandage. "This will help to retain the heat and relax the calf muscle so that it doesn't cramp up," he says. You can wear the combination wrap as long as it is comfortable.

Reach over the counter. To reduce the pain and inflammation of an injured calf, try an over-the-counter nonsteroidal anti-inflammatory drug (NSAID) such as ibuprofen, says Brent S. E. Rich, M.D., staff physician at Arizona Orthopaedic and Sports Medicine

Specialists in Phoenix and team physician at Arizona State University in Tempe. If you still need pain medication after a week, see a doctor.

Wear lifts. If your calf pain is caused by an injury, "take pressure off your heel," says Myles J. Schneider, D.P.M., a podiatrist in Annandale, Virginia, and co-author of *The Athlete's Health Care Book.*

Heel lifts (available at athletic shoe stores) can help ease the strain on tendons and muscles, says Dr. Selner. To make heel lifts, "cut two ¼-inch-thick pieces of cork and place them in your shoes."

Don't push it. Avoid any activity that puts undue stress on your calves—such as walking uphill or cycling—until your calf is completely healed, says John Cianca, M.D., assistant professor of physical medicine and rehabilitation at Baylor College of Medicine in Houston.

Squelch Cramps with Sensible Shoes

If your calf pain isn't the result of an injury, revamping your footwear may relieve the soreness, experts say. These shoe-shopping strategies can help.

Pamper your calves. Wear running shoes as often as possible, advises Dr. Selner. "If you have to wear dress shoes at work, change into them when you get to the office."

Toss those spikes. If you wear high heels, stop, recommends Dr. Selner. "Wear heels no higher than 1½ inches high." But if you're used to wearing very high heels, don't suddenly switch to flats: "The sudden change can trigger calf pain," he says.

Check your shoes' shocks. Replace worn shoes, says Dr. Schneider. "Losing the shock absorption in your shoes can lead to calf pain," he says. Once you lose ⅛ inch of tread, get new shoes or have the soles replaced.

Wear inner soles. These products, which are available in the foot-care section of any drugstore, can increase your shoes' shock absorption by 30 percent, says Dr. Selner.

Try arch supports. When you wear arch supports inside your shoes, they help correct mechanical imbalances that affect the way you walk. These imbalances may throw off your gait and put extra pressure on your calves, says Dr. Schneider.

Pain-Preventing Exercises

Stretching and strengthening the muscles in your calves can help prevent pain in the future, says Dr. Rich. Here's a simple routine to try. Just be sure to warm up your calf muscles, advises William S. Case, president of Case Physical Therapy in Houston. He suggests doing these exercises after you take a hot shower.

- Stand facing a wall and place your palms flat against the wall. Shift your stance to place one foot behind the other. Keep your back heel down and the toes of that foot turned slightly inward as you bend your front knee. Now lean into the wall, pressing it with your palms. Hold the stretch for 30 seconds.
- Sit on the floor with your legs straight in front of you, toes pointing upward. If you can reach your toes, grab them with your fingers and pull them toward you, stretching the calf. If you can't reach your toes comfortably, wrap a towel around your foot and pull on both ends to get the same effect. Hold for 30 seconds.
- Sit in a chair and raise and lower your heels. Or raise yourself up and down on your tiptoes, holding onto a table for support. Do one set of each exercise, starting with 20 repetitions and building up to 40 repetitions, says Case. But if you start to feel pain in your calves, stop and rest. "Don't exercise more than you're ready for," he says. "You may do more damage."
- Strengthening your shins may also reduce calf pain, adds Dr. Selner. Put 2 pounds of rice in a stocking and drape the stocking over your toes. Sitting in a chair with your knees bent and your feet on the floor, lean forward and pull your toes toward your shins. "This exercise strengthens the toe extensor muscle, so you put less pressure on the calf," he says.

Cancer Pain

Treating cancer pain depends on a variety of factors—the type of cancer you have, the extent of the disease, and your individual tolerance for pain. But while the source of the pain can vary, one thing is for certain: Most of the time, it can be controlled.

But you can't get relief if you don't ask for it, say experts. So it's crucial to let your family, doctors, and nurses know that you're hurting. "You're entitled to relief 24 hours a day, seven days a week, 52 weeks a year," says John D. Loeser, M.D., director of the Multidisciplinary Pain Center at the University of Washington in Seattle. Here is what you can do for yourself (and what doctors can do for you) to ensure your comfort.

Identify the Pain

Cancer pain can stem from physical factors—such as a tumor pressing on nerves or bone—or from side effects from treatments such as chemotherapy. It may also be aggravated by a whirlwind of overwhelming emotions such as anxiety or depression. The pain can be chronic (long-term and dull or intense) or acute (short-lived and intense).

To conquer the pain, say doctors, you have to identify it. Some experts suggest keeping a journal in which you jot down when the pain comes, where it hurts, how long it lasts, and its quality (sharp, throbbing, and so forth).

"Don't assume that your doctors know what you're feeling," says Sue P. Heiney, R.N., manager of psychosocial oncology at the Center for Cancer Treatment and Research of Richland Memorial Hospital in Columbia, South Carolina. "Anything you can tell them about your pain will help you get the best treatment for it."

Don't Go It Alone

Joining a cancer support group can mean the difference between suffering in silence and drawing strength from others, says Mark Goulston, M.D., assistant clinical professor of psychiatry at the University of California, Los Angeles, UCLA School of Medicine and author of *Get Out of Your Own Way.*

"There is a difference between pain and suffering," observes Dr. Goulston. "Suffering is often pain plus feeling alone with that pain. Cancer tends to make you feel very alone, which increases the sense of suffering."

When you join a support group, says Dr. Goulston, "you feel less alone because you're involved with people in the same struggle. Only people who are going through what you are can say 'I know how you feel' convincingly."

How You Can Help Yourself

The following strategies may help supplement the pain medication or other medical treatment that your doctor has prescribed. You'll most likely need assistance in putting these methods into practice, however. So ask your doctors to put you in touch with people who can help, including the experts at a cancer treatment center or pain clinic.

Honor your emotions. "Anxiety, depression, worry, fear—all of these emotions can influence how much pain affects you," says Dr. Loeser. "Recognize that these emotions play a role in the perception of pain and, if necessary, ask your doctor to refer you to a psychotherapist or counselor." You may also opt to join a cancer support group.

Take a stroll. Walk regularly, if possible, says Heiney. Even taking a brief walk around your room can improve your circulation and help your body metabolize pain medication, thereby controlling any side effects, she says.

Visualization for Pain Relief

This visualization exercise is recommended by Celeste Mills, a certified clinical hypnotherapist in Los Angeles and a spokesperson for the American Cancer Society.

1. Pick a time when you won't be disturbed. "Unplug the phone and ask family and friends not to bother you," says Mills.
2. Sit or lie down and close your eyes.
3. Take three deep, full breaths. "As you breathe in, imagine that you're taking in positive energy, health, and well-being," says Mills. "Then, as you exhale, imagine getting rid of toxins, stress, and negativity."
4. Conjure up an image of a healthy cell. "You may want to imagine it as a cartoon," says Mills. "To me, a cell looks like a Pac-Man–type character."
5. Imagine an army of healthy cells that you can dispatch to any part of your body. "Send" this army to the area where the cancer is located or where you may have undergone surgery. "See the tissue in that area becoming healthy and strong, like it was when you were a child," says Mills.

Perform this visualization for 10 to 15 minutes at a time at least once a day, or whenever you are feeling stressed, suggests Mills. "Think of this time as a pleasant, relaxing ritual," she says.

Exercise, if you can. Even gentle exercise can help release endorphins, your body's natural painkillers, says Avrum Bluming, M.D., a hematologist/oncologist and clinical professor of medicine at the University of Southern California in Los Angeles. "Get whatever exercise you can, within reason," he says.

Learn to relax. Stress-management techniques such as visualization and meditation may help reduce the sensation of pain, says Michael Ferrante, M.D., director of the program for cancer pain and symptom management at the University of Pennsylvania Medical

Center in Philadelphia. The most basic relaxation technique: Sit quietly and focus on your breathing for 5 to 10 minutes at a time. Or ask your doctor or nurse to recommend a relaxation audiotape.

Get a massage. Massage can help reduce emotional stress and thereby lessen your perception of pain, says Heiney. Massage can also relieve tight, tense muscles and help maintain your flexibility and range of motion, she says.

Try hypnosis. "Hypnosis has long been known to control pain," says Celeste Mills, a certified clinical hypnotherapist in Los Angeles and a spokesperson for the American Cancer Society.

Heiney concurs. "Hypnosis can help you dissociate from the pain," she says. "It's like turning down the dial from 10 to 2." You can find a qualified hypnotherapist through the American Society for Clinical Hypnosis. (You can write the Society at 2200 East Devon Avenue, Suite 291, Des Plaines, IL 60018.)

Heal your veins. To help ease tenderness and swelling caused by repeated injections, "apply aloe vera—straight from the plant, if possible—to the injection sites," says Mills. "Or make a paste out of goldenseal powder and water and pack it onto the affected areas before you go to sleep, leaving it on all night. Both treatments can help soothe the pain."

Try acupuncture. In acupuncture, special needles are inserted into the body at specific locations thought to control specific areas of pain sensation. "Acupuncture causes no harm, and it helps some people a lot," says Dr. Ferrante. A local medical association can put you in touch with qualified practitioners in your area.

Medical Options for Cancer Pain

Most cancer pain can be controlled with oral medication alone, says Dr. Ferrante. But if oral drugs don't help, there are other options that doctors can try.

"If your pain is acute, your doctor may give you intravenous

Write for More Help

For more information about treating cancer pain, contact the American Cancer Society's national resource center at 1-800-ACS 2345 (1 800 227 2345).

Also, the American Pain Society can send you a listing of pain centers in your area. For information, write to the organization at 4700 West Lake Avenue, Glenview, IL 60025.

---

medication, either intermittently or by a steady drip," says Dr. Bluming. Pain medication can also be administered by catheter into the spinal canal, he says. "This method may enable you to get by with less medication and fewer side effects."

Person-controlled analgesia is another increasingly popular—and empowering—way to manage pain, says Dr. Bluming. "Rather than lie in bed and buzz for a merciful nurse, you have pain medication in an IV bottle at your bedside," he says. You press a button to release the pain medication when needed. But because the medication is regulated automatically to give you increments preset by your physician, you can't give yourself more than what is safe, he says.

Many people tolerate more pain than they need to because they fear that they will become addicted to pain medication. Wrong, say experts. "There is no risk of addiction whatsoever," says Dr. Loeser. Many people who have cancer may develop a tolerance to medication, he says, meaning they need more of the drug to get the same relief. But if their doctors taper them off their medication correctly, they have no craving for the drug, he says.

Canker Sores

D on't let their size fool you. Canker sores, those tiny yellow or grayish-white ulcers that appear in your mouth without warning, pack a mighty painful punch. They turn simple acts such as talking and brushing your teeth into exercises in misery. Even eating becomes a torturous test of will.

Canker sores usually show up on the tongue, the floor of the mouth, or the inside of a lip or cheek. Experts don't know for sure what causes them. But research so far has pointed to a whole host of potential triggers—everything from a breakdown in the immune system to nutritional deficiencies, hormonal changes, abrasions and other minor mouth injuries, and even stress.

Squelch the Sting

If you develop a canker sore, it should clear up on its own within 10 to 14 days. In the meantime, you can do more than just wince and bear it. The following tips should help ease the pain.

Favor milder fare. When you have a sore, you'll instinctively avoid spicy and acidic foods such as chili and citrus fruits because of the pain they cause. That's exactly what you should do, according to Richard Price, D.M.D., clinical instructor at the Henry Goldman School of Dentistry at Boston University. Try to limit your diet to smooth, bland foods such as soft bread, scrambled eggs, and pasta.

Watch what you eat. "There are theories that canker sores may be caused by food allergies—in particular, to dairy and wheat products," says Thomas F. Razmus, D.D.S., associate professor in the

When to See the Dentist

Most canker sores will go away by themselves in two weeks or less, says Jay W. Friedman, D.D.S., a dental consultant in Los Angeles and author of *Complete Guide to Dental Health*. "But if the pain is acute and nothing you do relieves it, or if the sore persists, see a dentist," he advises.

department of diagnostic services at the West Virginia University School of Dentistry in Morgantown. Research has yet to offer proof of this dietary link. But if you have a tendency to develop canker sores, it can't hurt to eliminate dairy and wheat products from your diet to see if the sores stop occurring, he says.

Nix nicotine. Don't smoke when you're nursing a canker sore, says Howard S. Glazer, D.D.S., a dentist in Fort Lee, New Jersey, and past president of the Academy of General Dentistry. Nicotine can irritate the sore, which just fans the flames of pain.

Whip up some fast relief. Make a paste of baking soda and water, then dab a little on the canker sore, suggests Dr. Glazer. Use the paste as needed, but don't ingest it if you have high blood pressure.

Swish to soothe. Rinse your mouth with a liquid antacid as needed, suggests Barry C. Baron, M.D., associate clinical professor of otolaryngology at the University of California, San Francisco, School of Medicine. It will neutralize the acid in your mouth, thereby reducing the pain. "Liquid antacid is better than the chewable kind because the granules in a tablet can irritate a canker sore," he says.

Try acidophilus. There's some evidence that acidophilus—a beneficial bacterium found in yogurt—may help treat canker sores, says Melvyn Werbach, M.D., a physician in Los Angeles who special-izes in nutritional medicine and the author of *Healing with Food*. You will find acidophilus in liquid and tablet forms in most drugstores. Use the liquid as a mouthwash or let the tablets dissolve in your mouth with milk. Use either preparation four times a day, he recommends.

Think zinc. You may also want to consider taking 100 milligrams of zinc a day until the sore is healed, says Dr. Werbach. "Zinc supplements appear to be an effective treatment for canker sores, although this is not scientifically proven," he says.

Note: You should not take more than 15 milligrams of zinc a day without first consulting a physician.

Go over the counter. There are a variety of nonprescription medications for canker sores, such as Zilactin and Orajel, says Dr. Razmus. These products create a film "bandage" over a sore. Some also contain a numbing agent to temporarily block pain.

Carpal Tunnel Syndrome

What's the difference between Elton John and a computer operator? Victor Borge and a grocery-checkout clerk? Mozart and a needlepoint maven?

Give up?

Well, all the piano players are a lot less likely to get carpal tunnel syndrome (CTS). If we typed, price-scanned, or sewed the way piano players tickle the ivories—wrists straight, hands and fingers almost level with the keyboard—this debilitating wrist injury could often be prevented.

The carpal tunnel is a passageway that leads through your wrist. Nine tendons plus the median nerve—which feeds motor and sensory impulses to the thumb, index finger, third finger, and half of the ring finger—run through this tunnel of bone and ligament. If you have CTS, the tissues in this tunnel swell, compressing the median nerve.

This pressure means that the median nerve can't "translate" electrical impulses from the brain as well as it should. "Think of the median nerve as a radio or TV cable," says Larry Spitz, M.D., medical director of the Penn Diagnostic Center in Philadelphia. "If it stops sending a clear signal, you get static." Faulty signals from a compressed median nerve can cause tingling, numbness, and pain in the fingers, wrist, and even the forearm.

Many people think of CTS as an occupational hazard, caused by too much time at the computer. But any repetitive stress on the wrist—such as needlepoint, steady driving, and even golf—can trigger carpal tunnel syndrome. And continual wrist-twisting isn't the only culprit. The so-called passive form of CTS is caused by health conditions such as diabetes, thyroid disease, arthritis—even pregnancy.

When to See the Doctor

If you suspect that you have carpal tunnel syndrome, see a doctor immediately, say experts. If the condition is caught early enough, treatment may be as simple as wearing a splint or modifying habits that are aggravating the injury. If these remedies don't work, your doctor may recommend injecting corticosteroids into the carpal tunnel to reduce the swelling.

If steroid treatment doesn't help, you may need surgery, says David Rempel, M.D., associate professor in the division of occupational medicine at the University of California, San Francisco, School of Medicine. But surgery is considered the last resort, he says.

Taming the Tingling

If you have CTS, your doctor has most likely recommended that you stop or modify activities that involve repetitive wrist motion. But you can do more than keep the injury from worsening: You can reduce or stop the pain. Here's how to find relief.

Put the ache on ice. Fill a plastic bag with ice, wrap it in a thin towel, and vigorously rub it over the top of your wrist, suggests Leon Robb, M.D., director of the Robb Pain Management Group in Los Angeles. "The ice helps reduce fluid retention around the ligament that covers the carpal tunnel, which reduces the pressure on the median nerve," he says.

Keep your wrist in neutral. Wear a wrist splint, suggests John F. Lawrence, M.D., assistant professor of hand surgery at the University of California, Los Angeles, UCLA School of Medicine. You will find wrist splints in any drugstore.

Make sure that the splint you buy keeps your wrist absolutely straight, says Dr. Lawrence. "When you rest your splinted hand, palm up, on a table, it should lie flat, with your wrist in line with your forearm," he says. Wear the splint at night, too. Many people with CTS flex their wrists when they sleep, irritating the median nerves.

Try B$_6$. Take 50 milligrams of vitamin B$_6$ twice a day, suggests Dr. Robb. Some studies suggest that people with carpal tunnel syndrome tend to be deficient in this vitamin, which is associated with nerve function. "Some people with CTS can get dramatic relief with B$_6$," he says. "Nerves seem to respond to this specific vitamin, although we're not sure why."

Note: Consult your physician before taking this much vitamin B$_6$. High dosages of the vitamin can cause numbness in the feet and uncoordination when walking.

Reach for the sky. Keep your hands above the level of your heart as often as you can, says Ken Meadows, a physical therapist with the Portland Hand Rehabilitation Center in Portland, Oregon. Accumulated fluid in your hands can increase the pressure on the median nerve. "When you sit on your couch, for example, rest your elbows and hands on top of the backrest rather than keeping your hands in your lap," says Meadows. "Also, raise your hands two or three times a day for a few minutes to help prevent numbness and tingling."

Lose Weight—And the Smokes

Here is yet another reason to exercise, watch your diet, and stop smoking. People who smoke or are overweight are more likely to develop CTS, says James Stark, M.D., a physiatrist in the Center for Sport Medicine at St. Francis Memorial Hospital in San Francisco.

"Studies indicate that a couch potato will more frequently develop CTS than someone who is in good shape and of normal weight—perhaps because they tend to retain water," says Morton L. Kasdan, M.D., clinical professor of plastic and reconstructive surgery at the University of Louisville School of Medicine in Louisville.

Smoking can damage the median nerve as well. "Smoking causes blood vessels to constrict," Dr. Kasdan explains. "If the vessels that feed the nerve contract, it won't get enough circulation."

Chafing

You just bought a new shirt, and boy, are you irritated. No, it has nothing to do with the color, the size, or the fact that it's now on sale for 50 percent off. The collar has literally rubbed you the wrong way, leaving you with raw, red skin on the back of your neck.

Blame this painful patch on the friction that's created when fabric and skin come in contact. The constant rubbing causes chafing.

Though chafing is most likely to occur on the neck, some women experience it beneath their breasts, where a bra's elastic meets tender skin. The insides of the thighs can also become irritated when they rub against each other or against a pair of pants.

Save Your Skin

A case of chafed skin can make you miserable enough to want to burn your entire wardrobe. Fortunately, you don't have to resort to such drastic measures for relief. Here is what you can do to help heal your hurting hide—and protect it from future episodes of irritation.

Soothe the soreness. Apply an antibiotic ointment such as Neosporin to the affected area, advises Rodney Basler, M.D., a dermatologist in private practice in Lincoln, Nebraska.

Skip the petroleum jelly, though: "It can block the pores and aggravate chafing," says Jerome Z. Litt, M.D., assistant clinical professor of dermatology at Case Western Reserve University School of Medicine in Cleveland.

Take cover. "Covering the chafed spot can relieve much of your discomfort," says Joseph A. Witkowski, M.D., clinical professor of dermatology at the University of Pennsylvania School of Medicine

When to See the Doctor

Generally speaking, you can treat chafed skin on your own, says Jerome Z. Litt, M.D., assistant clinical professor of dermatology at Case Western Reserve University School of Medicine in Cleveland. Consult your doctor if the affected area is slow to heal, if it begins to ooze or weep, or if you have severe pain, particularly when you move, he advises.

in Philadelphia. He suggests using a thin, synthetic material called Spenco Second Skin, which is available in drugstores.

Keep it clean. Cleanse the affected area with a gentle, non-irritating soap such as Cetaphil, suggests Dr. Litt. You should avoid strong deodorant soaps, he says, because they can leave an irritating residue on the skin.

Loosen up. Avoid wearing tight clothing and abrasive fabrics when you have chafed skin, says David Margolis, M.D., assistant professor of dermatology at the University of Pennsylvania Medical Center in Philadelphia. He advises people who develop chafing around their necks to switch to the next larger collar size.

Examine your inseams. Don't wear pants with heavy inseams, especially when you exercise, says Dr. Litt. "Wear loose sports briefs or jogging pants made from satiny material," he says. "They'll diminish the friction between skin and fabric."

Take a powder. Dust areas that are prone to chafing with baby powder, suggests Dr. Litt. "Powder adds some slip to the skin and helps prevent rubbing," he says. Powder also absorbs moisture, which helps reduce friction.

Choose chafe-proof fabrics. If you are prone to chafing, avoid wearing clothes made from scratchy synthetic and woolen materials. Instead, opt for fabrics that breathe well, such as soft cottons.

Rinse well. When you do your laundry, be sure to thoroughly rinse the soap from your clothes, Dr. Witkowski advises. And don't use strong detergents or heavily perfumed fabric softeners, he says. These products can cause skin irritation and make chafing even worse.

Expose your skin. Chafed skin will heal faster if it's left uncovered and allowed to breathe, Dr. Litt says. While this may not be possible during the day, make sure that your sleepwear is loose and comfortable so that your skin can get some "airtime" while you snooze.

Childbirth Pain

Giving birth to a child can be one of the most joyful experiences of a woman's life, but it's undeniably one of the most painful. And the lingering controversy surrounding the role of pain medication during childbirth doesn't help matters. Should you opt for pain medication, or shouldn't you?

Answers vary, depending on whom you ask. Some experts believe that pain medication prevents a woman from fully participating in the birth of her child and may also harm the baby. Others believe that medication helps kill the pain while it keeps a woman alert and lowers the risk of fetal injury.

Whether you opt for pain medication is a personal decision that you need to discuss with your doctor early in your pregnancy, says Emanuel Fliegelman, D.O., professor emeritus of obstetrics and gynecology and director of the human sexuality program at the Philadelphia College of Osteopathic Medicine. But whatever you decide, you owe it to yourself to know all of your options.

Being Prepared Can Ease the Pain

Being physically and emotionally ready for childbirth can significantly reduce a woman's perception of pain, experts agree. That is why many doctors recommend that mothers-to-be and their partners take a course in prepared childbirth (such as the Lamaze method). The goal of this approach to labor and delivery is to educate both parents-to-be for the upcoming birth.

The benefits of taking such a class can be considerable: a shorter labor and less trauma during labor and delivery. "These classes can help educate you about what to expect, so it's not all new and

---

| **What the Doctor Can Do** |

The most common medical option for pain relief during childbirth is the epidural.

In an epidural, doctors inject a small amount of a numbing drug near the spine. "Epidurals can provide virtually complete relief from labor pain," says Mark Norris, M.D., professor of anesthesiology, obstetrics, and gynecology and chief of the section of obstetric anesthesiology at Washington University School of Medicine in St. Louis. Serious side effects are rare. Moreover, the pain medications used today allow a woman to avoid the pain while still being alert and "present" during the delivery.

You should know, however, that some doctors believe that epidurals slow labor and increase the risk of cesarean delivery. Dr. Norris admits that anesthesia during delivery remains controversial. Your best bet is to "discuss your options with your obstetrician and anesthesiologist well before you go into labor," he says.

---

frightening," says Mark Norris, M.D., professor of anesthesiology, obstetrics, and gynecology and chief of the section of obstetric anesthesiology at Washington University School of Medicine in St. Louis. "There is a correlation between prenatal anxiety and the amount of pain during labor. The more anxious a woman is, the more pain she tends to experience."

One study seems to confirm Dr. Norris's experience. Sixty women evaluated their performance during childbirth for a researcher at the University of South Carolina College of Nursing in Columbia. Twenty-seven of these women reported "managing well" during labor and delivery and said that understanding what was happening during childbirth helped them stay in control.

Learning relaxation techniques such as deep breathing also seems to help lessen childbirth pain. Studies show that pregnant women who practice these techniques for 30 minutes during the day have quicker, easier labors, according to Nancy Marshutz, R.N., a nurse-midwife at the Natural Childbirth Institute and Women's Health Center in Los Angeles. Some women practice self-hypnosis as they are giving birth, and experts agree that it can provide some—if not complete—pain relief.

Consider a Midwife

Women who opt for natural childbirth often choose to deliver with the help of a certified nurse-midwife. Certified nurse-midwives use a variety of natural methods to help a woman manage childbirth pain, such as visualization, self-hypnosis, massage, and soothing lighting and music.

"If a birth proceeds normally, most women don't need pain medication," contends Marshutz. "But if they do, there is always the option of going to the hospital." If you opt for natural childbirth, however, you should know that anesthesia may be required if you need a cesarean section.

Cold Sores

Like canker sores, cold sores (also known as fever blisters) can hurt like the dickens. But that's where the similarity ends. Unlike canker sores, cold sores are caused by a virus—the herpes simplex virus—and usually erupt outside rather than inside your mouth. One more thing: Cold sores are highly contagious.

Most people acquire the herpes virus in childhood. And most of the time, this silent invader lurks unnoticed in your system, only to flare up when you're under emotional stress, when your resistance is low, or even when you've been exposed to too much sun. You'll first feel a burning, itching, tingling, or numbness around the area. Then, you'll develop a small blister that ruptures and forms a crust. Voilà: a full-blown cold sore.

Speedy Relief for Cold Sores

The pain of a cold sore tends to fade during the first few days, and the sore itself is usually history within 7 to 10 days. But you can ease a sore's sting and speed the healing process with these tips.

Have some cold comfort. As soon as you feel the telltale tingling, warning you that a cold sore is coming on, "wrap an ice cube in a washcloth and hold it directly on the tingling spot," says Melvyn Werbach, M.D., a physician in Los Angeles who specializes in nutritional medicine and the author of *Healing with Food*. Ice the area two or three times a day for 15 to 20 minutes at a time. Remove the cube every 2 minutes for about 15 seconds.

Keep the sore moist. Dab the cold sore with a lip ointment such as Blistex several times a day, says Richard Price, D.M.D., clin-

When to See the Doctor

If your cold sore doesn't clear up within 10 days, see a doctor, says Richard Price, D.M.D., clinical instructor at the Henry Goldman School of Dentistry at Boston University. Because there's a small risk of cancer, "any sore in or around the mouth that doesn't go away in a week to 10 days should be examined."

ical instructor at the Henry Goldman School of Dentistry at Boston University. "Don't let a cold sore get too dry," he says. "It can crack, which can delay healing and increase the pain."

Pat on some E. Prick a vitamin E capsule and squeeze some of the contents onto your cold sore, says Dr. Werbach. "Vitamin E may speed the healing of wounds in the moist mucous membranes of the mouth," he says.

Zap the pain with zinc. Apply zinc sulfate ointment to a cold sore every hour when it first appears, and then several times a day after that, says Dr. Werbach. "In preliminary studies, zinc sulfate stopped the pain of a cold sore within 2 to 3 hours," he says. "And regular use of the zinc greatly reduced the chance of the sores coming back."

Lick blisters with lysine. For an acute outbreak of cold sores, take 1,000 milligrams of the amino acid lysine three times a day, says Dr. Werbach. You'll find lysine supplements in the vitamin sections of drugstores or health food stores. "Studies have shown that taking lysine supplements can reduce the severity and frequency of outbreaks," Dr. Werbach notes. Once the blisters have healed, take 500 milligrams a day to prevent a recurrence, he says. Consult with your doctor, however, before you take this supplement. In some people, "lysine can cause the liver to step up its production of cholesterol," he warns.

Get some Zs. Dab a cold sore with an over-the-counter mouth-pain ointment such as Zilactin-B, suggests Dr. Price. "These products are effective, although Zilactin-B contains alcohol, which can sting."

Keep the cap on the steroids. Never use a topical steroid on a cold sore, says Thomas F. Razmus, D.D.S., associate professor in the department of diagnostic services at the West Virginia University School of Dentistry in Morgantown. "Topical steroids can cause the herpes virus to spread," he explains.

Bye-Bye Fever Blisters

Of course, there's something even better than pain relief for a cold sore, and that's prevention. Here's what you can do.

Screen your kisser. Shield your lips with sunscreen, says Dr. Price. "Studies show that the use of sunscreen can make a big difference." He recommends using a product with a sun protection factor (SPF) of 15 or more.

Learn to relax. Practice relaxation exercises to calm your body and reduce outbreaks, says Dr. Werbach. "Stress can cause the herpes virus to emerge from hiding."

Don't poke or pick. To stop a cold sore from spreading, keep your hands off it, says Howard S. Glazer, D.D.S., a dentist in Fort Lee, New Jersey, and past president of the Academy of General Dentistry.

Stop the spread. To keep your family safe, too, you need to guard against common forms of infection. Wash your hands carefully before you touch your eyes or genitals. Anyone with cold sores should use separate silverware, drinking glasses, toothbrushes, and washcloths.

Avoid arginine. If you are prone to cold sores, avoid peanuts, chocolate, cereal grains, gelatin, carob, and raisins, says Dr. Werbach. These foods contain an abundance of the amino acid arginine, which promotes the growth of the virus.

Pop some vitamin C. Take 500 milligrams of vitamin C twice a day, suggests Dr. Werbach. "Many studies have shown that vitamin C can help fight viral infections," he says. "Supplementation might give your immune system an extra boost."

Corneal Burns and Abrasions

The two most common causes of burns to the cornea, which sits over your iris and pupil like the crystal on a watch, are sun exposure and contact with common household chemicals.

The *strangest* cause of corneal burns? Curling irons.

You read right: This unlikely injury can happen when a woman is curling her bangs—but the curling iron slips, burning her eye, says Jay Lustbader, M.D., assistant professor of ophthalmology at Georgetown University School of Medicine and director of the Cornea Center, both in Washington, D.C. A corneal burn can cause scaring pain: It's been described as the feeling of sand in your eyes.

And then there's what doctors call a corneal abrasion—a scratch on the surface of your cornea caused by an errant speck of mascara or by falling asleep without removing your contact lenses. A corneal abrasion will make your eye red, painful, and teary; it may even affect your vision.

Fortunately, the cornea is remarkably resilient, says Deborah Banker, M.D., an ophthalmologist in Boulder, Colorado, who specializes in natural vision improvement. "The outer layer of cells on the cornea are among the fastest healing tissues in the body," she says. But make no mistake: You can't neglect an eye injury, no matter how minor it seems.

Get Aid ASAP

The simplest way to prevent corneal burn, say eye experts, is to wear sunglasses whenever you are outdoors. The shades you choose

When to See the Doctor

Any eye injury—including a corneal burn or abrasion—should be examined by a doctor, says Jay Lustbader, M.D., assistant professor of ophthalmology at Georgetown University School of Medicine and director of the Cornea Center, both in Washington, D.C.

Also, an abrasion should be examined by an eye doctor to make sure that the break in the cornea does not get infected, says Deborah Banker, M.D., an ophthalmologist in Boulder, Colorado, who specializes in natural vision improvement.

should block 100 percent of ultraviolet (UV) rays and should be large enough to keep UV rays from getting under, over, or around the frames. ("And keep your curling iron away from your eyes," adds Dr. Lustbader.)

But if you should burn or abrade your cornea (or sustain any type of eye injury), don't rely on self-help remedies to kill the pain: Be sure to get to an eye doctor as quickly as possible, advises Dr. Lustbader.

Here are some suggestions for what you should do until you can get to an eye doctor's office.

Make like a pirate. If you burn or scrape your cornea, "wear a cotton patch over your eye until you can get to a doctor," advises Dr. Lustbader. Or you can simply roll up a piece of gauze and tape it over your eye. Wearing a patch will help keep your eyelid from rubbing against your cornea, he explains. "Keeping your eye closed won't eliminate the pain completely, but it will diminish it significantly," he says.

Flush out your eye. If you are splashed in the eye with a chemical, you should immediately flood the eye with cool water for at least 15 minutes, recommends the American Academy of Ophthalmology. Hold your head under a faucet or shower or gently flush out your eye with water from a clean container, while rolling your eyeball around as much as you can. Use your fingers to keep your eye wide open.

Keep your eye moist. As your eye heals, "Keep it well lubricated with artificial tears at night," advises Dr. Banker. "You can aggravate an abrasion when you open your eyes in the morning." Don't forget to use artificial tears during the day as well.

Corns

Take a good look at the toes of any woman who frequently wears high heels. Chances are, you'll see a corn on each little toe—painful reminders of a certain weakness for exquisite but ill-fitting shoes.

Corns are made up of layers of dead skin that form on the bony parts of the foot, especially the toes. Your skin sprouts these painful bumps to protect itself from pressure. There are two varieties of corns: hard and soft. Hard corns, which usually form on the little toe, are caused by repeated friction. Soft corns, which form between the toes, are most often caused by wearing narrow shoes that crowd the toes.

Pain-Proof Those Toes

Soft or hard, corns are no walk in the park. Here's how to pain-proof your crop of corns.

Soak, then file. Soak a hard corn in warm water until it's soft—which usually takes about 15 minutes. Then file the corn gently with a pumice stone, says Rock Positano, D.P.M., co-director of the Foot and Ankle Orthopedic Institute at the Hospital for Special Surgery in New York City. "Make sure that you don't file the tender skin underneath and around the corn," he says. Afterward, slather the corn with mineral oil or moisturizer.

Pad the painful corn. Shield hard corns with corn pads—doughnut-shaped pads that fit around the corn and protect against pressure and friction, says Dr. Positano.

Give soft corns some space. To ease the pain of soft corns, separate your toes with cotton or lamb's wool, suggests Carol

Frey, M.D., a foot and ankle surgeon at the Orthopedic Hospital in Los Angeles. Or use a toe separator, available in the foot-care section of any drugstore.

Pass on corn plasters. Avoid using corn plasters and other over-the-counter corn removers, says Dr. Positano. "Many of these products contain salicylic acid, which can burn or injure the tender skin under the corn if they're not applied properly," he says. It's especially important to avoid these preparations if you have diabetes or poor circulation, he says. That's because an acid burn may heal very slowly or even become infected—and you could have reduced sensation in your toes if you have these conditions.

Wear the Shoes That Fit

Rule one for corn control: Wear properly fitting shoes. "You should be able to freely wiggle all of your toes," says Dr. Frey. "There should be ½ inch between the end of your longest toe, which is not necessarily the big toe, and the end of the toe box." These other tips can help, too.

Toss those stilettos. Switch from narrow, spiked heels—which can crowd the toes and cause soft corns—to walking pumps, which have a wider toe box and more manageable heels. "You'll find plenty of comfortable, attractive walking pumps," says Dr. Frey.

Shop late. Buy new shoes at the end of the day when your feet are largest, advises Dr. Frey.

Please rise. "Get fitted while you're standing, not sitting down," says Dr. Frey. That's because your feet spread slightly when you're standing, so you'll be sure to get a larger size shoe.

For the same reason, always get a shoe size that accommodates your larger foot. "Most people have one larger than the other," Dr. Frey notes.

Study your shoes and socks. "See if your shoe is excessively worn or if it has a torn seam or lining," suggests Glenn Gast-

When to See the Doctor

If nothing you do soothes the pain of your corn, see a doctor or a podiatrist. He may prescribe orthotics—foot supports worn inside your shoes to correct your gait. Especially stubborn corns may require surgery, but it's a minor procedure.

wirth, D.P.M., deputy executive director of the American Podiatric Medical Association. Check your socks or stockings, too; a tear in a seam can cause friction, as can wadded-up hose.

Don't peel your corns. *Never* pare away a corn with a razor blade, says Dr. Gastwirth. This is especially important if you have reduced sensation because of poor circulation or diabetes, he says. "You might not feel pain very well and may not realize how much you have injured yourself," he says.

Cuts and Scrapes

An unpleasant encounter with a kitchen knife. An embarrassing stumble during your daily constitutional. A too-close shave with a razor blade. All manner of everyday activities can leave you with the unkindest cut (or scrape) of all

No matter how thick-skinned you are, these minor injuries hurt. Their small size often belies the pain they can cause. Still, you probably won't win much sympathy for your agony when what you're sure is a mortal wound turns out to be nothing more than a paper cut.

Actually, any pain you experience is a good thing. It reminds you to take care of that cut or scrape pronto. And that's important, experts say, because any open wound—even a small one—is an open invitation to infection caused by bacteria.

Fast Fixes for Minor Ouches

When one of life's little mishaps leaves its mark on your skin, prompt first-aid can ease any discomfort and help speed healing. Here is what the experts say that you should do.

Stem the flow. Compression not only stops the bleeding but also helps reduce the pain, says Libby Bradshaw, D.O., assistant professor of family medicine and community health at Tufts University School of Medicine in Boston. She suggests applying firm pressure directly over the injury with a clean cloth for 5 to 10 minutes. The blocked blood flow exerts pressure on the pain fibers, so you feel pressure rather than pain, she explains.

Keep it clean. Flush a cut or scrape with running water to help remove dirt and debris, says David Margolis, M.D., assistant pro-

---

Getting Out of a Sticky Situation

Sometimes the hurt of a cut or scrape is no match for the agony of removing an adhesive bandage. To keep the procedure as pain-free as possible, experts recommend using a fingernail scissors to separate the gauze from the adhesive part of the bandage. Cut along either side of the gauze and lift it from the wound. Then gently pull the adhesive strips from your skin.

If the scab is sticking to the gauze, soak the area in a salt-water solution (about 1 teaspoon of salt for each quart of water). The dressing will loosen on its own.

---

fessor of dermatology at the University of Pennsylvania Medical Center in Philadelphia. Cleansing the wound is vital to reduce the risk of infection.

Don't forget to dress. Apply an antibiotic ointment to the cut or scrape, then cover it with an adhesive bandage or a piece of gauze. Besides keeping the wound clean and protected, the dressing is also likely to ease pain, says Dr. Bradshaw. "It will remind you that the cut or scrape is there, so you're less likely to bump it," she notes. Leave the wound uncovered at night so that it can breathe, she adds.

Say hello to aloe. An old standby as a treatment for burns, aloe vera is great first-aid for cuts and scrapes as well. The cool, colorless gel seals off the wound, relieves pain, and speeds healing. Simply break a leaf off an aloe vera plant and squeeze the leaf's contents onto your cut or scrape; apply the gel three or four times a day for maximum benefit.

Go Krazy. "The neatest thing in the world for a paper cut is an instant glue (such as Krazy Glue)," says Rodney Basler, M.D., a dermatologist in private practice in Lincoln, Nebraska. "Apply it directly to the cut twice a day. It immediately seals off the cut and stops air from hitting the nerve endings, which is what causes the pain."

When to See the Doctor

An extremely deep or wide cut should be examined by your doctor, says Libby Bradshaw, D.O., assistant professor of family medicine and community health at Tufts University School of Medicine in Boston.

Also see your doctor if you develop any sign of infection such as a fever, streaky red lines leading away from the wound, or pus, says Jack Rudick, M.D., professor of surgery at Mount Sinai School of Medicine of the City University of New York in New York City.

Ask your doctor whether you might need a tetanus shot, especially if the cut has been exposed to dirt or bacteria and you haven't had a shot in five years, says Dr. Bradshaw.

If you don't happen to have the glue on hand—or if you are wary of using it—try petroleum jelly instead. "It protects exposed skin tissue from the air," says Dr. Basler. "And the moisture helps new tissue to grow."

Hands off. Once a cut or scrape forms a scab, leave it alone, says Jack Rudick, M.D., professor of surgery at Mount Sinai School of Medicine of the City University of New York in New York City. Besides being painful, picking away a scab is picking away protection. "A scab is nature's way of putting a dressing on a wound," he says. "If you pick at it, the wound may reopen, and the healing process will have to start all over again."

Denture Pain

E ver wonder why George Washington had that perpetually sour countenance—the one we know so well from our grade-school history books and the one-dollar bill? Maybe it was because those wooden dentures were killing him.

Dentures have come a long way since the Father of Our Country sported his wooden choppers. But denture pain is still with us. "Ill-fitting dentures can feel like a pebble in your shoe," says Kenneth M. Hargreaves, D.D.S., Ph.D., associate professor in the divisions of endodontics and pharmacology at the University of Minnesota Medical School in Minneapolis.

When pain starts, the first step should be to contact your dentist. Most dental pain can be traced to a denture plate that needs to be recast or remade. In fact, "dentures usually have to be refitted every three to four years," says Amerian Sones, D.M.D., a dentist in private practice in Santa Monica, California.

If you think that you can grin and bear it, better reconsider. Sores on the mouth or gums that are constantly irritated by dentures can lead to more serious problems, says Howard S. Glazer, D.D.S., a dentist in Fort Lee, New Jersey, and past president of the Academy of General Dentistry.

Hints for Happy Gums

The bottom line is: If your dentures hurt, see your dentist. But until your appointment, try these pain-away tips.

Soften up your diet. Whether you're breaking in new dentures or having trouble with older choppers, choose easy-to-chew food, says Dr. Sones. "For the first week or so that you have new dentures,

When to See the Doctor

If a mouth sore lingers for more than 10 days, see a doctor. "Be particularly wary of a painless mouth sore," says Jay W. Friedman, D.D.S., a dental consultant in Los Angeles and author of *Complete Guide to Dental Health.* The constant irritation of a dental plate against your gums can lead to cancer, he says.

Also see a doctor if you have pain when you tighten your jaw, find it difficult to open your mouth, or "click" when you open and close your mouth, recommends Ira Klemons, D.D.S., Ph.D., director of the Center for Head and Facial Pain in South Amboy, New Jersey. You may have temporomandibular disorder, a condition that affects the jaw joint.

avoid crusty breads and tough meats," she says. "Stick to soft foods such as pasta, rice, ground meat, and poached fish."

Go without. If your dentures are extremely painful, don't wear them until you can see your dentist, suggests Dr. Sones. While this may not be an option if you have to go to work or attend meetings, maybe you can take a day off or postpone appointments until the problem is fixed.

Put your dentures back in an hour or so before you see the dentist, "so that he can see exactly what's causing the irritation and where," says Dr. Glazer.

Massage away the pain. "A minute-long gum massage every day will help toughen up the tissue, which makes a stronger base for dentures," says Dr. Sones. The Academy of General Dentistry suggests grasping your gums between your thumb and fingers or gently brushing your gums with a soft- or extra-soft-bristle toothbrush, using a circular motion.

Give your gums a bath. Swish your mouth with a saltwater rinse—1 teaspoon of salt to 1 cup of warm water, suggests Dr. Sones. (Be sure to spit out the rinse rather than swallowing it.)

Try OTC relief. Rub your sore gums with an over-the-counter topical painkiller (such as Orajel), suggests Dr. Sones. But don't use this medication for too long: "It can irritate the tissue," she advises.

Keep Those Juices Flowing

Is your mouth as arid as the Sahara? A dry mouth can make denture pain worse, says Richard Price, D.M.D., clinical instructor at the Henry Goldman School of Dentistry at Boston University.

To keep your whistle wet, carry a bottle of water with you, says Dr. Sones. Or suck on sugar-free lozenges to keep your mouth moist. But beware: The sorbitol in sugar-free lozenges can cause gas, diarrhea, and bloating in some people.

Some medications—including antidepressants, antihistamines, and drugs for heart problems, high blood pressure, and eye conditions—can cause dry mouth. Your doctor may be able to change your medication, says Thomas F. Razmus, D.D.S., associate professor in the department of diagnostic services at the West Virginia University School of Dentistry in Morgantown. But if not, "at least you'll know the source of the problem."

Diverticulosis

If your diet has come up short in the roughage department over the years, you may notice the effects sometime after your 60th birthday. That's usually about the time pea-size pouches called diverticula start to form in the walls of the intestines, most often in the lower part of the digestive tract.

Sixty-five percent of us will have developed diverticula—a condition called diverticulosis—by the time we turn 85. "Like gray hair, diverticula come with age," says Marvin Schuster, M.D., former director of the division of digestive diseases at Johns Hopkins Bayview Medical Center in Baltimore.

Diverticulosis usually doesn't hurt. In fact, most people don't even know they have it until the telltale pouches show up on an x-ray or during an intestinal exam.

For an unlucky 10 to 25 percent of those with diverticulosis, though, the condition worsens to diverticulitis. This means that the usually benign pouches become infected and inflamed, causing rectal bleeding, constipation, and severe abdominal pain. Between 15 and 30 percent of people with acute diverticulitis require surgery.

Defend Yourself against the Big D

Clearly, diverticulitis is serious business. But you can do a lot to put a pox on those pouches and keep an *-osis* from turning into an *-itis*. For starters, try the following tips.

Feast on fiber. Diverticula are usually a by-product of eating too much highly processed, low-fiber fare. Getting more fiber in your diet minimizes the likelihood that diverticula will form in the first place, says Walid H. Aldoori, M.D., adjunct professor of epidemiology

When to See the Doctor

Diverticulosis seldom requires medical attention, experts say. But severe pain in the lower left part of your abdomen or a change in your usual bowel habits—perhaps accompanied by rectal bleeding, constipation, or fever—may indicate the onset of diverticul*itis*. These symptoms are your cue to get to your doctor immediately, says Walid H. Aldoori, M.D., adjunct professor of epidemiology at the School of Medicine at Memorial University of Newfoundland.

in the School of Medicine at Memorial University of Newfoundland.

Even if you already have diverticulosis, eating fiber-rich foods can help by relieving the constipation that is often a symptom of the condition. "Fiber dilates the colon and reduces the pressure inside it," Dr. Aldoori explains.

Among the best food sources of fiber are fruits, vegetables, and whole-grain breads and cereals. Add these to your diet slowly to minimize the gas pain that often accompanies an increase in fiber intake. (Any discomfort that you do notice should only be temporary, experts say.) According to nutrition guidelines established by the U.S. Department of Agriculture, you should aim for at least 25 grams of fiber per day. Don't get hung up on numbers, though. Just eat a whole-grain or bran cereal at breakfast, such as granola or bran flakes. Choose a whole-grain bread at lunch and add fresh fruits and vegetables to each meal.

Note: If you have acute diverticulitis, you should avoid high-fiber foods. "In that case, you want to rest the bowel," says Roger Gebhard, M.D., professor of medicine at the University of Minnesota in Minneapolis.

Don't be seedy. Stay away from foods that contain small seeds, including tomatoes and popcorn, and dishes prepared with whole-seed spices such as cumin and sesame, says Naurang Agrawal,

M.D., professor of medicine at the University of Connecticut School of Medicine in Farmington. "The seeds can lodge in the diverticula and cause inflammation," he explains.

Banish red meat from your plate. "We've found that the higher the intake of red meat, the greater the risk of diverticular disease," says Dr. Aldoori. Neither chicken nor fish appears to produce a similar increase in risk, he notes.

Drink plenty of water. "Fluid makes the contents of the gut moister and lessens the pressure inside the colon, which may be responsible for the formation of diverticula," Dr. Aldoori says. Try to drink at least eight 8-ounce glasses of water a day.

Get moving. The more active you are, the less likely you are to develop diverticular disease, says Dr. Aldoori, who led a study that examined the link between exercise and diverticular disease in 47,678 men. "The best results, in terms of reduced risk, were associated with vigorous activities such as jogging and racquet sports," he says.

Try tranquillity. When it comes to your digestive health, it's not only what you eat but how you eat that's important, says Brian Rees, M.D., medical director of Maharishi Ayur-Veda Medical Center in Pacific Palisades, California. His suggestions: "Take meals without stress or distraction, never eat while standing up (you are not relaxed while standing), and observe a moment of silence before eating—say a prayer or just close your eyes for a moment."

Ear Pain

If the last time you had an ear infection was back in the second grade, consider yourself lucky. While most of us do get our earaches out of the way in childhood, there are times when adults get them. One bad cold can trigger ear pain that can make even a grown-up cry.

Ear pain comes in other forms besides earaches, such as swimmer's ear and "airplane ear." And sometimes what you think is ear pain can be traced to problems with your mouth, teeth, jaw, throat, or sinuses. So the first thing that you have to do is figure out what's up. Here are some of the possibilities.

"Airplane ear." The bane of frequent (or any) fliers, this ache occurs when the eustachian tube, which runs between your mouth and middle ear, can't equalize the change of atmospheric pressure. A vacuum is created inside your ear—and that pulls at your eardrum, triggering pain.

Ear pain that isn't. Your "ear pain" may actually be caused by a dental condition, a sinus infection, neuralgia (a sharp pain in a nerve or group of nerves), or the aching-jaw condition known as temporomandibular disorder.

Middle-ear infection (otitis media). Children are most likely to develop this kind of ear pain. But adults can develop these infections, too, especially when they have bad colds. You most likely have a middle-ear infection if you feel pressure deep in your ear—like you're talking in a tunnel—if you swallow and you hear water pop or you can't clear your ear, says Barry C. Baron, M.D., associate clinical professor of otolaryngology at the University of California, San Francisco, School of Medicine.

Swimmer's ear. This painful condition starts when water gets stuck in the ear canal, which creates an ideal breeding ground for fungus and bacteria. First, your ear feels blocked and itchy, but soon it becomes red, tender, and swollen.

Soothing Strategies for Any Ear Pain

Ear infections usually don't go away on their own, says Thomas J. McDonald, M.D., chairman of the department of otolaryngology/head and neck surgery at the Mayo Clinic in Rochester, Minnesota. So when you have ear pain, it's wise to see an ear, nose, and throat specialist (oto-laryngologist). Until you do, here are some ways to get relief.

Keep your head high. Sit up rather than lie down, says Dr. McDonald: "Reclining can make ear pain worse," he explains.

Apply a warm pack. Wring out a washcloth in warm (not hot) water and place it over your ear, says Dr. McDonald. Apply the packs for 10 to 15 minutes every 2 hours. You might also place a cotton ball that has been soaked in warm water into the little crevice between the earlobe and ear opening.

Drop in some drops. Warm some mineral oil or baby oil and, using an eyedropper, gently drop the oil into your ear canal, says Dr. Mc-Donald. Don't use drops if you see or feel drainage from your ear, he says. "Drainage is actually a good thing," he explains. "It means that your eardrum has ruptured and the pus can drain. Seeing your ear drain can be a bit alarming, but the pain is relieved, and you'll feel better quickly."

Go for the garlic. When you have ear pain, eat a clove or two of garlic a day, says Julian Whitaker, M.D., founder and president of Whitaker Wellness Center in Newport Beach, California. "Garlic has natural antiviral and antibiotic qualities that kill many of the germs that cause earaches," he says. If you're not a fan of fresh garlic, try garlic supplements, available in most health food stores and many drugstores.

When to See the Doctor

If self-help remedies don't ease your ear pain or if you develop drainage from your ear or any loss of hearing, see a doctor, says William H. Slattery, M.D., an otolaryngologist at the House Ear Clinic in Los Angeles.

Also see a doctor if the pain gets progressively worse even when you have been prescribed antibiotics, if it gets worse when you drink a hot beverage, or if you have difficulty swallowing. These symptoms can signal a more serious condition, says Thomas J. McDonald, M.D., chairman of the department of otolaryngology/head and neck surgery at the Mayo Clinic in Rochester, Minnesota.

If your doctor can't find anything wrong with your ear, consider seeing a doctor or dentist who specializes in head and facial pain, says Ira Klemons, D.D.S., Ph.D., director of the Center for Head and Facial Pain in South Amboy, New Jersey. This is especially important if you have any of the following symptoms: headaches, facial pain, eye pain, blurry vision, dizziness, pressure or ringing in the ears, or difficulty swallowing. The American Academy of Head and Facial Pain can refer you to a specialist in your area. Send your request and a self-addressed, stamped envelope to the academy at 520 West Pipeline Road, Hurst, TX 76053-4924.

Also see a doctor if you have pain when you tighten your jaw, find it difficult to open your mouth, or "click" when you open and close your mouth, recommends Dr. Klemons. You may have temporomandibular disorder, a condition that affects the jaw joint.

Reach for pain relief. Take an analgesic such as Extra Strength Tylenol, suggests Dr. McDonald. "An over-the-counter pain reliever can help you to feel more comfortable until you can see a doctor."

Easing Swimmer's Ear

The first time that you get swimmer's ear may be your last, if you follow the tips below.

Fight bacteria or fungi with vinegar. Using an eye-dropper, drop 6 to 10 drops of an equal mix of distilled white vinegar and water into your ear, suggests William H. Slattery, M.D., an oto-laryngologist at the House Ear Clinic in Los Angeles. "The ear canal is usually a little acidic," he explains. "An infection causes the canal to lose some of that acidity and encourages bacteria to grow. The vinegar rinses help restore this acidity and can help prevent an ear infection from worsening."

Avoid these rinses if you know that you have a perforated eardrum, see or feel drainage from your ear, or develop any loss of hearing, adds Dr. Slattery.

Oil up. If you are prone to swimmer's ear, drop mineral oil or baby oil into your ears *before* your swim, says Dr. McDonald.

Blow-dry your ears. After a swim, hold your hair dryer several inches from your ear and dry out your ears, suggests Dr. Slattery. "The temperature should be comfortable—not too hot," he says.

Try rubbing alcohol. To help prevent swimmer's ear, place a drop or two of rubbing alcohol into your ear within an hour after you swim, advises Dr. Slattery. "The alcohol will dry out your ear canal but may cause your ears to itch," he says. Don't use alcohol if you have a perforated eardrum, see or feel drainage from your ear, or develop any loss of hearing, he says.

Coping with "Airplane Ear"

Do your ears crackle more than a container of Rice Krispies when you fly? Try this strategy, suggests Dr. McDonald.

Before your flight, buy some gum and an over-the-counter nasal spray. "As you taxi down the runway, chew the gum, close off one nostril, spray decongestant into the other, and swallow some saliva at the same time," says Dr. McDonald. Then spray your other nostril. "This method is almost guaranteed to work," he adds. Use the same technique just before you're ready to land.

Note: Don't use a decongestant if you have a heart disorder or an abnormal pulse.

Also, try to delay your nap until the plane reaches cruising altitude, says Dr. Slattery. "When you sleep, you don't clear your eustachian tube as frequently as you do when you're awake," he explains.

Endometriosis

For most women, the menstrual period is just a fact of life, a monthly occurrence as unremarkable as sending in a car payment. Not so for women with endometriosis.

In endometriosis, the tissue that lines the uterus, called the endometrium, implants and grows in areas it shouldn't. This wandering tissue sometimes bleeds and/or secretes an irritant into the surrounding tissue when a woman gets her period. So she is hit with cramps and pain wherever the tissue has implanted—which could be the outside of the uterus, the ovaries, fallopian tubes, bladder, or bowel. But the pain is not necessarily associated with the menstrual cycle; it can occur at any time.

Endometriosis pain affects women differently, depending on where the tissue has implanted. Symptoms may include painful periods and bowel movements, lower back pain, and pain during sex. For some women endometriosis can be associated with infertility and heavy or irregular bleeding.

It's crucial to diagnose endometriosis as soon as possible, says David Redwine, M.D., director of the Endometriosis Institute in Bend, Oregon. "Women are often told by well-meaning people—their mothers, sometimes even their doctors—'This pain is just a normal part of being a woman.' That kind of attitude can lead to a delay in the diagnosis, which results in unnecessary pain—because the pain gets progressively worse."

You *Can* Ease the Pain

Endometriosis is virtually impossible to cure short of surgery. But there is a variety of ways that you can get relief.

When to See the Doctor

If you have severe pelvic pain before and during menstruation or experience heavy or irregular bleeding, be sure to see a doctor, say experts. You should also consult your doctor if you have painful bowel movements or urination, pain during intercourse, or lower back pain.

"If your pelvic pain causes you to miss work or otherwise limits your activities, see a doctor. Don't waste time thinking that the pain will go away," says David Redwine, M.D., director of the Endometriosis Institute in Bend, Oregon.

While endometriosis is the most common cause of pelvic pain in women, "it's often diagnosed as another condition such as a pelvic infection, an ovarian cyst, or ovulation pain," he adds. "The first thing to rule out is endometriosis. So if your doctor doesn't raise the possibility, raise it yourself."

Soothe with heat. Place a warm heating pad on your abdomen, says Dr. Redwine. "Keep the temperature comfortably warm, and use the pad as long as you need to," he says. (As extra insurance against burns, you should put a cloth between the pad and your skin.)

Try an oil pack. Cover your abdomen with a castor-oil pack, advises Christiane Northrup, M.D., assistant clinical professor of obstetrics and gynecology with the University of Vermont College of Medicine at the Maine Medical Center in Portland, Maine. Here's how: Soak a piece of flannel in cold-pressed castor oil and place it over your lower abdomen, directly on your skin. Cover the cloth with a hot-water bottle and lie on your back for an hour. "The castor oil gets into your lymph nodes and may help your immune system remove implanted endometrial tissue," says Dr. Northrup. You can find cold-pressed castor oil at health food stores.

Try to keep moving. While there's no evidence that exercise will help cure endometriosis, "there is evidence that women who exercise are less likely to have this condition," says Dr. Redwine.

If you're in too much pain for vigorous exercise, "try strength training, riding a stationary bike, or another activity that doesn't jostle you around too much," suggests Lisa Rarick, M.D., director of the division of reproductive and urological drug products at the Food and Drug Administration. If the pain is severe, she says, "at least try to ex ercise before your period—it may help reduce your discomfort."

Drink lots of water. Drink eight 8 ounce glasses of water a day, says Dr. Rarick. Water retention can increase endometriosis pain, and the more fluid you take in, the less likely you are to retain water.

Skip the moo food. Cut back on processed dairy foods such as milk, cheese, and yogurt, recommends Dr. Northrup. "My clinical experience has shown that nonorganic dairy foods increase estrogen levels," she says—and that increase can intensify the pain.

Modify meat eating. Limit your consumption of red meat to 6 ounces or less, three times per week. Red meat is high in arachidonic acid, which can lead to tissue inflammation. Instead, try to eat at least 2 cups of cruciferous vegetables (such as broccoli and cauliflower) a day, along with 20 to 50 grams of soy protein (about one-third of a block of tofu), suggests Dr. Northrup. In addition, have at least ½ cup of cooked whole grains such as barley or brown rice.

Get your B vitamins. Take a multivitamin/mineral supplement that contains 50 to 100 milligrams of each of the B vitamins, suggests Dr. Northrup. "The B vitamins can help your liver process estrogen more effectively," she advises.

Eat more fish. Consume more fish high in omega-3 fatty acids such as mackerel, salmon, and tuna, says Dr. Redwine. "There is some evidence that a diet high in fish oil can help reduce endometriosis pain. Fish oil is thought to stimulate the good type of prostaglandin, which doesn't cause pain, instead of the bad type, which causes inflammation." Or opt for fish oil capsules, taken according to the dosage on the label.

Try natural progesterone. Massage ¼ to ½ teaspoon of a nonprescription natural progesterone cream (such as ProGest) into the soft areas of your skin three times a day, alternating between your face, neck, inner thigh, inner arms, and breasts, recommends Dr. Northrup. "Natural progesterone helps counteract the effects of excess estrogen," she explains. If you have pain only after ovulation, start the cream just before you ovulate and continue through your period, she says.

Don't confuse natural progesterone cream with the yam-derived creams usually sold in health food stores, Dr. Northrup says. You'll want a product with a 3 percent formulation. If it's not available in your area, you can order it by mail from Transitions for Health, 621 S.W. Alder Street, Suite 900, Portland, OR 97205-3627.

Go the OTC route. Take an over-the-counter nonsteroidal anti-inflammatory drug (NSAID) such as ibuprofen or aspirin, says Dr. Rarick. Any nonprescription pain reliever should be taken as directed, so read the label or ask your pharmacist about dosages.

What a Doctor Can Do

Your doctor may prescribe one of a variety of drugs to treat endometriosis. "Oral contraceptives can help lessen endometrial pain before and during menstruation," says Dr. Rarick.

A doctor may also prescribe the steroid derivative danazol (Danocrine) or one of a class of drugs called GnRH agonists. GnRH agonists, which are similar to the natural brain hormone gonadotropin-releasing hormone (GnRH), interfere with ovulation and menstruation. Side effects of danazol sometimes include hot flashes, weight gain, irregular vaginal bleeding, lowering of the voice, and facial hair. The GnRH agonists have all the side effects of menopause, including an increased risk of developing osteoporosis, heart disease, hot flashes, and joint pain. These symptoms are not permanent because the drug is only taken for six months, explains Dr. Northrup.

If endometriosis is severely advanced or painful, many doctors recommend laparoscopic surgery. In this procedure, a surgeon inserts a telescope-like device called a laparoscope through a small incision in the abdomen and removes endometrial tissue by zapping it with a laser or by actually cutting it away.

Eye Pain

Y ou rub your left eye. Five minutes later, you rub it again. Pretty soon, you're pawing your peeper like a mutt with an itch he can't reach. A look in the mirror reveals that the white of your eye has turned a flamboyant scarlet. What gives?

Almost anything, unfortunately. Your eyes can be irritated by foreign matter, from a speck of dust to an errant fleck of mascara. They may itch or burn, irritated by allergies, dirty contact lenses, or too many hours spent unblinking in front of your computer. Maybe you got socked in the eye with a tennis ball or lightly thwacked with your niece's or nephew's plastic Power Ranger.

Or, for one reason or another, your eyes may not produce enough tears, leading to the stinging, burning, and grittiness of dry eye.

You may even have developed conjunctivitis (also called pinkeye), a bacterial or viral infection of the membrane that lines the eyelid and covers the eyeball. Or maybe you have a sty, an infection of one of the oil glands in the eyelid.

Other possible causes of eye pain include blepharitis, which is an infection of the eyelids, and inflammation caused by allergy. Either of these can turn your baby blues or browns into red, tender puffs.

The first thing to do: Stop pawing. The second thing: Try some of the following pain-easing tips.

Relief for Raw Orbs

How you ease eye pain depends on what's causing it in the first place. Cold compresses, hot packs, artificial tears, homemade eye washes, and a host of other self-treatments can go a long way toward soothing red, irritated peepers.

When to See the Doctor

See an eye doctor if you have severe pain in or around your eye, says Jay Lustbader, M.D., assistant professor of ophthalmology at the Georgetown University School of Medicine and director of the Cornea Center, both in Washington, D.C. "You may think you have a headache, but it may be glaucoma," he says. Pain that is accompanied by blurred vision or discharge from your eye also requires medical attention.

Another reason to schedule an appointment with an eye doctor is your eyes becoming extremely sensitive to light, says John Sheppard, M.D., associate professor of ophthalmology at the Eastern Virginia Medical School of the Medical College of Hampton Roads in Norfolk. "You may have an infection, a cataract, or corneal disease."

But if you sustain a serious eye injury, or what you thought was a minor injury doesn't heal within a few days, don't rely on self-help remedies to kill the pain, cautions Jay Lustbader, M.D., assistant professor of ophthalmology at Georgetown University School of Medicine and director of the Cornea Center, both in Washington, D.C. Get to an eye doctor as quickly as possible. In the meantime:

Irrigate your eye. To dislodge any speck of dust or grit "wash out your eye with saline solution, preferably one without preservatives," says Deborah Banker, M.D., an ophthalmologist in Boulder, Colorado, who specializes in natural vision improvement. Don't use tap water, distilled water, or eyedrops unless you have splashed your eye with a caustic chemical and there is nothing else available, says Michael B. Raizman, M.D., associate professor of ophthalmology at Tufts University School of Medicine in Boston.

Dab away the invader. If the fleck or speck is on the white part of your eye, try to dislodge it—*gently*—with a damp cotton swab, says Dr. Lustbader.

Flip your lid. Another way to dislodge a painful particle is to pull your upper lid down over the lower lid, says John Sheppard, M.D., associate professor of ophthalmology at the Eastern Virginia Medical School of the Medical College of Hampton Roads in Norfolk. "Pulling down your lid will allow the foreign body to wipe off on the skin of the lower lid so you can dislodge it," he says.

Give dry eyes the cold treatment. To ease dry eyes, apply a bag of crushed ice or ice cubes to the affected eye for 5 minutes every 2 hours, says Dr. Sheppard.

"Or use a cold egg right out of the refrigerator," says George N. Dever, O.D., an optometrist in private practice in Seattle who practices holistic and traditional eye care. Just take the whole egg (with the shell intact) and gently press it against your sore eye.

Make yourself "cry." To combat dry eye, bathe your eyes with artificial tears, says Dr. Lustbader. "These products mimic real tears," he says. They are available at most drugstores.

Put the pain on ice. If you get socked in the eye, experts suggest immediately applying an ice pack to your eye for 15 minutes. Cold can reduce the pain and swelling.

Speedy Relief for Sties and Pinkeye

The first symptoms of a sty are teariness, sensitivity to light, and the feeling that something is in your eye. Then the lid reddens, swells—and hurts. A sty is a low-grade infection of the eyelid, says Dr. Lustbader.

For quick relief, place a washcloth soaked in warm water over the sty for 15 minutes every 2 hours, says Dr. Raizman. "The compress will liquefy the oils and allow them to drain," he says. "This treatment will cure most sties." What *not* to do? "Don't rub your eye and don't wear eye makeup," he says.

To ease conjunctivitis, rinse your eyes with an eyewash made from 1 teaspoon of salt and 1 pint of boiled water, writes Charles Thomas, Ph.D., a physical therapist at Desert Springs Therapy Center in Desert Hot Springs, California, and co-author of *Hydrotherapy: Simple Treatments for Common Ailments.* Cool the mixture before you put it in your eye. Repeat this treatment every few hours.

You can also take a 30C dose of Apis, a honeybee venom extract, once or twice a day until your eye begins to feel better, says Judyth Reichenberg-Ullman, a doctor of naturopathy and co-author of *The Patient's Guide to Homeopathic Medicine.* (The notation 30C refers to the remedy's potency, which is indicated on the label.) You'll find Apis in health food stores.

Eyestrain

With apologies to moms everywhere, it's time to set the record straight: You won't ruin your eyesight by reading in dim light. "Eyestrain as the cause of vision problems is an old wives' tale," says John Sheppard, M.D., associate professor of ophthalmology at the Eastern Virginia Medical School of the Medical College of Hampton Roads in Norfolk. "Your eyes are designed to be used 24 hours a day."

Still, staring at computer and television screens for hours on end can tax your eye muscles and make your eyes water and sting. Unfortunately, your baby blues (or browns or greens) weren't built to handle the visual bombardment delivered by these modern-day emitters.

But technology shouldn't take all the blame for eyestrain. You can get it from driving a car, from exposure to air pollution, and from reading all that fine print on pill bottles, car ads, and credit card statements.

Respite for Sore Eyes

The pain of eyestrain can affect more than your eyes. At times you may feel it spread to the rest of your head or to your neck or back.

Thankfully, a little R and R is all it takes to perk up pooped peepers. Here's what the experts advise.

Listen to your eyes. Give your eyes a rest when they need one, experts say. The pain won't go away unless you give up the offending activity—at least for a little while.

Be inclined to recline. "Lie down in a dark room with a hot compress over your eyes," suggests George N. Dever, O.D., an op-

When to See the Doctor

Eyestrain responds quite well to self-care and seldom requires medical attention, experts say. Nevertheless, you should see your doctor if you experience piercing or throbbing eye pain, blurred vision, or an extreme sensitivity to light.

In the case of chronic eyestrain, you may want to consult an optometrist. He may prescribe eyeglasses as a preventive measure—even if you have 20/20 vision, says Susan C. Danberg, O.D., an optometrist in private practice in Glastonbury, Connecticut.

"Suppose you work at a computer a lot and you're experiencing discomfort or fatigue," she says. "Eyeglasses can reduce the burden on your eyes. They help you focus so that your eyes don't get so tired."

tometrist in private practice in Seattle who practices holistic and traditional eye care. To make the compress, simply soak a towel or washcloth in water that is as hot as you can stand.

Make some heat. A technique called cupping can ease eyestrain, according to Oscar Janiger, M.D., associate clinical professor at the University of California, Irvine, School of Medicine and author of *A Different Kind of Healing*. "First, rub your hands together to make them warm," he says. "Then gently press your palms against your closed eyes and hold them there for a while. You'll find it very soothing."

Orbit your orbs. Using your thumb or forefinger, gently press the bone surrounding each eye socket, Dr. Dever says. "Start at the upper inner corner of your eye and move along the top of the bone toward the outer corner of your eye," he explains. "Then move along the bottom of the bone toward your nose." Press each point along the way for 10 to 20 seconds.

Look distant. When you are working up close, remember to shift your focus every 30 minutes or so, experts say. "Try to look out

---

Revitalize Computer Eyes

You can reduce eyestrain when working on a computer by heeding this advice from Susan C. Danberg, O.D., an optometrist in private practice in Glastonbury, Connecticut.

Space yourself. Put some distance between you and the computer screen. "The screen should be 21 to 24 inches away from you, with the focal point (the text you're reading, for example) slightly lower than eye level," she notes.

Be flat-footed. When you're seated at a computer, your chair should be adjusted so that your feet rest flat on the floor. "If your body is in a bad position, then your eyes are in a bad position," she points out.

Eliminate glaring problems. Glare from a window or a lightbulb can contribute to eyestrain. If you can't move your computer, then shield the screen with either a hood or a glare screen. And keep the screen clean by wiping it from time to time with an antistatic cloth.

---

more than 20 feet," advises Michael B. Raizman, M.D., associate professor of ophthalmology at Tufts University School of Medicine in Boston. "Doing that for 1 to 2 minutes allows the muscles of your eyes to relax."

Exercise your eyes. To prevent eyestrain, Dr. Dever recommends what he calls eye yoga. His instructions: Move your eyes slowly and smoothly as far to the left as you can, then as far to the right as you can. Continue by looking up, then down, then at all four diagonals. Repeat the entire sequence three to five times, once or twice a day. You may feel a little pain at first, he says. Stop if it's too much.

Have passion for Ping-Pong. "Watching table tennis gives your eye muscles a good workout," Dr. Janiger says. "You move your eyes from side to side as well as up and down." If you can't find any live action, there is always the table tennis scene in *Forrest Gump*.

Read right. "Don't read when you're lying down—especially on your side," says Susan C. Danberg, O.D., an optometrist in private practice in Glastonbury, Connecticut. "When you're on your side, one eye is closer to the page than the other, so you get unequal focusing." Instead, hold the book parallel to your face. "If your head is tipped forward, for example, the book should be tipped slightly back," she advises.

Get illuminated. Adequate lighting is important to preventing eyestrain. But you also want to be sure that you have the right kind of lighting. "Avoid high-intensity lamps," Dr. Danberg suggests. "They cast shadows and cause glare." Opt for incandescent lamps instead. "Put one on each side of you so that you get equal brightness with no shadows," she says.

Take time-outs. Allow for a short break at least every ½ hour to give your eyes a well-deserved rest, Dr. Raizman suggests. "You learn from experience how often you need to take a break," he says. Just remember that the idea is to stop eyestrain before it starts.

Have your eyes examined. If you wear glasses and experience eyestrain, you may need a new prescription, says Jay Lustbader, M.D., assistant professor of ophthalmology at the Georgetown University School of Medicine and director of the Cornea Center, both in Washington, D.C. "You can easily overwork your eye muscles if your eyes need correction and don't get it," he explains.

Facial Pain

When your back went out of whack, you blamed it on spring cleaning—an entire weekend of hauling boxes from the attic to the basement. And when your knees knocked with pain, you could trace it to that afternoon you spent crawling around your garden planting petunias. But what could make your face hurt?

In reality, just about anything. "Facial pain has a variety of causes," says Ira Klemons, D.D.S., Ph.D., director of the Center for Head and Facial Pain in South Amboy, New Jersey.

Your face may hurt because of a sinus infection, a dental problem, a migraine, an allergy, or stress. Food additives such as monosodium glutamate (MSG) can trigger facial pain as well.

Perhaps the best-known source of facial pain is temporomandibular disorder, or TMD. In this condition, the temporomandibular joint—which connects the lower jaw to the temporal bone on the side of your head—becomes misaligned or inflamed. (For a more detailed discussion of TMD, see the chapter on page 255.)

Less well known is the condition known as trigeminal neuralgia, or tic douloureux. The pain follows the path of the trigeminal nerve on either side of the face—and it's excruciating. "It's probably the most severe pain known to humans," says Dr. Klemons.

Facing Off against Pain

Because such a wide array of underlying problems can produce facial pain, zeroing in on the exact cause usually requires the help of a doctor. In fact, more severe cases may require input from a whole team of medical professionals, including a family physician, a dentist, an otolaryngologist, and a neurologist.

When to See the Doctor

Facial pain has so many possible causes that it's best to have a doctor diagnose the underlying problem, experts say. "If your pain lasts for more than a day or two, get professional help," advises Samuel Seltzer, D.D.S., professor emeritus of endodontology at the Temple University School of Medicine and Dentistry in Philadelphia. Here are some symptoms to watch for.

- Pain when you bend over
- A feeling of "heaviness" in the face
- Nasal stuffiness, discolored mucus, or postnasal drip
- Difficulty opening your mouth
- Pain when you compress your jaw
- Clicking sounds when you open and close your mouth

And get to an emergency room immediately if you have weakness, numbness, or paralysis in your face, if you're vomiting, or if you're unable to turn your head, says Ira Klemons, D.D.S., Ph.D., director of the Center for Head and Facial Pain in South Amboy, New Jersey.

Even though you may need expert assistance to help you find the source of your pain, you can do a lot on your own to relieve your immediate discomfort. Here's what experts suggest for pain relief.

Make nice with ice. Massage the affected area with a cold pack or a plastic bag filled with ice cubes until the area is numb, suggests Leon Robb, M.D., director of the Robb Pain Management Group in Los Angeles. "For pain in your forehead, apply the ice to the back of your neck, just below your skull," says Dr. Robb. "For pain across your face, apply the ice just above your jawbone." Lay a thin towel over the affected area so that the ice doesn't make direct contact with your skin.

Limit your treatment sessions to no more than 10 minutes of every hour, Dr. Robb cautions. Leaving the ice on longer than that could make the pain worse.

Give peas a chance. If you don't have a cold pack handy or you're out of ice cubes, use a bag of frozen peas instead, suggests Steven Syrop, D.D.S., director of the TMD–facial pain program at Columbia University School of Dental and Oral Surgery in New York City. "The bag will adapt to the contours of your face," he notes.

Heal with heat. If muscle tightness is causing your discomfort, apply moist heat (such as a warm towel) to the painful area for about 15 minutes at a time, recommends Dr. Robb. You can do this five to six times a day.

Hit the spot. You can also relieve a muscle spasm by applying gentle pressure in the area of the facial nerve, says Dr. Robb. The point is located at the jaw joint, just in front of each ear and right below the cheekbone. You can feel it when you open and close your mouth. Steadily press the point on the affected side with your finger for 1 to 2 minutes, keeping your mouth closed, he says. Repeat as often as necessary.

Treat yourself to a mini-massage. Pain in your forehead may originate in the back of your neck, says Dr. Robb. "Massaging the back of your neck, just below your skull, may bring relief," he says.

Stave off stress. "Stress doesn't cause facial pain, but it can make it worse," says Dr. Klemons. Consider learning a relaxation technique that you can use during tense times such as meditation, visualization, or yoga.

Pick a painkiller. A nonsteroidal anti-inflammatory drug (NSAID) can provide relief, especially if you have trigeminal neuralgia. Try an over-the-counter medication such as aspirin or ibuprofen.

Get the point. Acupuncture is highly effective in easing facial pain, says Irwin Koff, M.D., a general practitioner in Kahuku, Hawaii, who is certified in acupuncture. "The procedure has no side effects if it's performed properly," he notes. He suggests contacting a qualified acupuncturist in your area. To find one, call your local hospital's physician referral service.

Fissures and Abscesses

Oh, the indignity. Of all the parts of your body, it would have to hurt . . . you know, down there. You may find little comfort in the fact that you don't necessarily have a hemorrhoid. But you should know that your anal pain is more likely the result of a fissure or an abscess, according to Max M. Ali, M.D., director of Hemorrhoid Clinics of America in Oak Park, Michigan.

What's the difference? A hemorrhoid is essentially a varicose vein of the anus or rectum. (For a more detailed discussion of hemorrhoids, see the chapter on page 138.) A fissure, on the other hand, is a small tear in the lining of the anal canal. If that tear becomes infected, you could develop an abscess.

No matter which affliction has aggravated your anal area, you can mostly likely blame it on constipation. As you have unwittingly discovered, trying to pass a hard, dry stool can do lots of damage to the tender tissues of your throbbing bottom.

Soothe Your Sit-Upon

Except in the most serious cases, a fissure or an abscess will heal on its own with time and a little tender loving care. You can help it along by following this advice from the experts.

Sit in a sitz. A warm sitz bath can provide fast, temporary relief from anal pain, Dr. Ali says. His instructions: Fill your bathtub with 6 to 8 inches of water that is between 85° and 95°F. Then sit in it and soak for about 10 minutes. Repeat at least three times a day, he suggests.

Wipe wisely. Don't be too rough when you clean the anal area after a bowel movement, advises John A. Flatley, M.D., retired clinical

When to See the Doctor

If a fissure doesn't go away on its own or if it keeps coming back, you should see your doctor, says John A. Flatley, M.D., retired clinical instructor of surgery at the University of Missouri—Kansas City School of Medicine. A chronic fissure may require surgery.

An abscess can be much more serious than a fissure, particularly if it is located in the rectum. Because feces are present at the site of the abscess, it may need to be drained.

A doctor's visit is also advisable any time you experience persistent anal pain, a significant change in bowel habits, or blood in your stool—especially if you are over age 40 and it's happening for the first time, says Max M. Ali, M.D., director of Hemorrhoid Clinics of America in Oak Park, Michigan.

instructor of surgery at the University of Missouri—Kansas City School of Medicine. Aggressive hygiene can irritate the area even more. "Try moistening the toilet tissue before you wipe, so it's not as abrasive," he suggests.

Lighten the load. Use an over-the-counter stool softener containing docusate sodium (such as Ex-Lax stool softener or Doxidan) so that you have less anal pain when you move your bowels, Dr. Ali says. If you have high blood pressure and are trying to limit your sodium intake, however, check with your doctor or pharmacist for a product that's right for you.

Ease the way with an enema. Constipation not only causes fissures and abcesses but aggravates them once they occur. You can relieve constipation with an enema, says Oscar Janiger, M.D., associate clinical professor at the University of California, Irvine, School of Medicine and author of *A Different Kind of Healing*. "Use about two glasses of warm water in a standard enema bag," he advises. "It's easier on the anus than a laxative."

Forage for fiber. Increasing your fiber intake makes the stool soft and less irritating to the anus, says Dr. Ali. He recommends eating more fresh fruits and vegetables and less cheese and red meat.

Stay well-hydrated. A hard, dry stool means that you're not getting enough fluids, Dr. Flatley says. To soften it up, he advises drinking at least six 8-ounce glasses of water a day. "I drink two glasses of water first thing in the morning, before breakfast, and I keep drinking water all day long," he notes.

Check your medication. "Codeine and its derivatives can cause severe constipation," Dr. Ali says. If you need a pain reliever, ask your doctor or pharmacist to suggest an over-the-counter anti-inflammatory. Such products don't contain codeine.

Foot Pain

The average person walks about 100,000 miles—the equivalent of four times around the Earth—over the course of a lifetime. And every single step along the way exerts hundreds of pounds of pressure on the feet.

With a workout like that, your "dogs" are entitled to do a little barking once in a while.

Actually, for all the wear and tear they endure, your feet hold up surprisingly well. Their complex construction (each foot has 26 bones, 33 joints, and more than 100 tendons, muscles, and ligaments) makes them quite sturdy and flexible. They have to be: "Your feet are your body's shock absorbers," notes Rock Positano, D.P.M., co-director of the Foot and Ankle Orthopedic Institute at the Hospital for Special Surgery in New York City.

Despite their ingenious design, there is one form of punishment that your feet simply can't withstand: the wrong shoes. According to the American Academy of Orthopaedic Surgeons, ill-fitting footwear is the primary cause of foot pain. Interestingly, most complaints of foot pain come from women, who account for more than 80 percent of all podiatric surgery patients. A study conducted by Carol Frey, M.D., a foot and ankle surgeon at the Orthopedic Hospital in Los Angeles, revealed that 88 percent of women wear shoes at least one width size too small and that 80 percent have foot pain related to their shoes.

Help for Hurting Feet

Unfortunately, many people wrongly believe that foot pain is normal—part of the price humans have to pay for walking upright. "Foot pain isn't necessarily caused by something serious," notes Glenn

Shoe-Shopping Savvy

Podiatrists agree that the best thing you can do to ease foot pain is throw out your cruel shoes and select a new pair on the basis of comfort rather than style. Here are their suggestions for finding shoes with the perfect fit.

- Shop for shoes at the end of the day, when your feet are at their largest.
- Don't choose shoes simply by "your size" alone. One manufacturer's size 8 may be another's size 7½.
- Fit shoes standing up rather than sitting down.
- Have the clerk measure both of your feet. For most people, one foot is bigger than the other.
- Make sure there's ½ inch between the end of your longest toe and the end of the shoe's toe box. (Your longest toe isn't necessarily your big toe. It is often your second toe.)
- If you wear insoles or orthotics, put them in when you try on shoes.
- Make sure the shoes are comfortable the moment you put them on. You should not have to stretch the shoes or break them in.
- When you try on shoes, walk in an area that is not padded and carpeted. Also, walk around for a while—don't take just two or three steps.
- If you're a woman who must wear heels, don't go any higher than 2¼ inches. And make sure that the toe box of the shoe is round rather than pointed and wide enough to move your toes.

Gastwirth, D.P.M., deputy executive director of the American Podiatric Medical Association. "But like any other pain, it's your body's way of telling you that something isn't right and needs attention."

The good news is, a little pampering can go a long way in helping your feet feel better. Here's what the experts advise when your dogs are hounded by pain.

Take a load off. It may seem obvious, but it bears repeating: "If your feet hurt, try to stay off them," says Dr. Positano. "Do a minimal amount of walking—or even better, don't walk at all."

Put them on ice. To reduce any swelling, apply ice to your feet for 15 to 30 minutes, three or four times a day, Dr. Positano suggests. "Use a disposable ice bag or a reusable ice unit that you freeze, like the ones for picnic coolers." Whichever you choose, be sure to wrap it in a towel to protect your skin from damage.

Soak in scented water. "When your feet ache, soaking them in water can be very refreshing," says Dr. Positano.

Aromatherapists often recommend adding 10 drops each of juniper and lavender essential oils to 2 quarts of cold water, then soaking your feet for 10 minutes. Essential oils are available in health food stores.

Stay cool. Don't use heat to ease your aching feet, Dr. Positano cautions. "Heat causes more swelling. Applying cold is your first line of defense."

Give them a lift. Elevating your feet can help reduce any swelling, Dr. Positano says. He recommends raising them 6 to 8 inches above your heart—especially while you sleep. Use pillows for more comfort.

When to See the Doctor

It's a good idea to see a podiatrist or an orthopedist who specializes in foot and ankle problems if you experience any of the following, says Rock Positano, D.P.M., co-director of the Foot and Ankle Orthopedic Institute at the Hospital for Special Surgery in New York City.

- Your pain lasts more than a week.
- Your pain seriously limits your activities.
- Your foot appears to be infected.

Offer much-kneaded relief. "Massaging your feet stretches the tissues and increases circulation," says Dr. Gastwirth.

Here's a simple self-massage suggested by Elliott Greene, past president of the American Massage Therapy Association.

Sit in a comfortable chair and cross your left foot over your right leg. Oil your fingers, if needed, with vegetable oil or massage oil. Glide the tip of your thumb up the middle of your sole, from the back of your heel to the base of your toes. Repeat on the right side of your sole, then on the left side. Then switch feet. You should spend about 2 minutes on each foot.

Next, retrace all three lines on your left foot by pressing from your heel to the base of your toes with the tip of your thumb. Then gently rub and squeeze your toes. Repeat on your right foot. You should spend 3 to 4 minutes on each foot.

Don't lose your marbles. Dr. Frey suggests this exercise to soothe tired, aching feet: Lay 20 marbles on the floor, then pick up each one with your toes and drop it into a small plastic bowl. "I suggest plastic because it muffles the sound of the marbles dropping into the bowl," she says. "That way, you can do the exercise in your office, seated at your desk." Aim for at least one session a day, she adds.

Seek some sole support. If your feet constantly ache, consider wearing insoles, Dr. Gastwirth says. "They're especially helpful in shoes with thin soles, like deck shoes. They make your feet feel much better." You can purchase insoles in drugstores and many sporting goods stores.

Consider orthotics. The next step above insoles is orthotics, which require a doctor's prescription. Unlike insoles, orthotics not only comfort aching feet but also help correct podiatric problems, Dr. Gastwirth says. "Orthotics reduce the strain on muscles that are working overtime to compensate for poor body mechanics."

Take a break from shoes. You know how much better you feel when you slip out of your shoes at the end the day. Your feet appreciate it, too. "The human foot was designed to be bare," Dr. Frey says. "So kick off your shoes whenever you can."

Gallbladder Pain

In most cases, gallstones are painless. In fact, you usually find out that you have them while undergoing a routine checkup or an exam for another illness.

But when gallstones act up—*ouch!* You may feel sudden, severe pain in the upper abdomen that can last from 20 minutes to several hours. That's the result of a stone as small as a speck or as large as an egg getting wedged in the duct that leads from the gallbladder into the intestine.

Sometimes the pain will radiate to your back and shoulders. And once you have a gallstone attack, you're likely to have another.

What causes these little nuggets of pain?

In a nutshell, the problem arises from the way that you metabolize cholesterol. Your liver produces bile, a cholesterol-rich fluid that your body uses to digest fats. Bile is stored in the gallbladder. Too much cholesterol in your bile can form soft clumps that eventually harden into stones.

As unfair as it seems, women are three times as likely as men to develop gallstones because females have more hormones racing through their systems. It's thought that the female sex hormones progesterone and estrogen may affect the amount of cholesterol in bile as well as the functioning of the gallbladder.

Tame Those Stones

There's no instant relief for gallbladder pain. But you *can* take steps to keep gallstones as docile as possible. Here's how.

Defat your diet. Reduce your intake of dietary fat. "If you have gallstones, consumption of fat, especially animal fat, may trigger

When to See the Doctor

If you experience nausea, vomiting, or severe pain in your right upper abdomen, see your doctor, says Sidney F. Phillips, M.D., professor of medicine at the Mayo Clinic in Rochester, Minnesota.

If you have gallstones that aren't causing pain (called non-symptomatic gallstones), the best treatment is to do nothing, says Dr. Phillips. For more troublesome gallstones, many doctors suggest laparoscopic surgery. Using a flexible, telescope-like device called a laparoscope, a surgeon can first see the gallstone and then remove it through a small incision in the abdomen.

gallbladder spasms," says Melvyn Werbach, M.D., a physician in Los Angeles who specializes in nutritional medicine and the author of *Healing with Food.*

Once you have gallstones, dietary changes alone will not get rid of them. "But eating less fat can help minimize the risk of symptoms appearing," says Rodger A. Liddle, M.D., chief of gastroenterology at the Duke University Medical Center in Durham, North Carolina.

Shed extra pounds. Try to maintain your ideal weight, experts advise. "People who are overweight are at a much higher risk for developing gallstones," says Xavier Pi-Sunyer, M.D., professor of medicine at Columbia University and director of endocrinology and nutrition at St. Luke's/Roosevelt Hospital Center, both in New York City.

Nix the crash or fast. If you need to lose weight, do so gradually, says Dr. Liddle. "Overweight people who go on extremely low calorie diets or who fast for days or weeks tend to develop gallstones," he says.

Also, don't consume a totally fat-free diet. "Have one meal a day with at least 10 grams of fat," says Dr. Pi-Sunyer.

Eat breakfast. People who skip breakfast are essentially undergoing a short-term fast, and fasting has been shown to increase the risk of gallbladder disease.

See if you're C-deficient. Ask your doctor if you may be deficient in vitamin C or hydrochloric acid (a component of gastric juice), advises Dr. Werbach. "Studies indicate that animals with a high-cholesterol diet and vitamin C deficiency are prone to developing gallstones. Another study found that about half of all people with gallstones are deficient in hydrochloric acid."

If your doctor finds that you have either deficiency, you can take steps to correct it, Dr. Werbach says.

Gas Pain

You're eating low-fat cheese and calcium-rich skim milk. Munching platefuls of fresh greens. Scarfing bowlfuls of beans. You're eating right and feeling virtuous.

You're also feeling as though a symphony is playing the *1812 Overture* in your guts. One big difference, though. Gas isn't just musical. It's downright painful.

But don't feel bad: A healthy diet is a gaseous diet, says Sidney F. Phillips, M.D., professor of medicine at the Mayo Clinic in Rochester, Minnesota. "Foods that are good for us, such as fiber, generate gas," he says.

That said, it must also be admitted that there are also less benign causes of gas. Other possible causes include lactose intolerance, an "allergy" to lactose, which is the sugar in milk and other dairy products; the artificial sweetener sorbitol; and swallowing air while you eat or drink.

Fast Relief for a Delicate Dilemma

No matter why you have gas, you undoubtedly feel motivated to get rid of it, preferably in the most graceful way possible. While the quickest path to relief is to let it out, so to speak, that's not always possible. These tips may help relieve your discomfort.

Keep a food diary. Write down what you're eating for a week or so, suggests David Peura, M.D., associate professor of medicine at the University of Virginia Health Sciences Center in Charlottesville. "See what you are eating on good days and gassy days," he says.

The most likely suspects are foods that contain sugars, espe-

---

When to See the Doctor

If your gas doesn't go away within a week or is accompanied by cramping, a change in bowel habits, sudden weight loss, or rectal bleeding, see a doctor, says Naurang Agrawal, M.D., professor of medicine at the University of Connecticut School of Medicine in Farmington. If you see blood in the stool that's bright red, it's probably a sign of rectal bleeding. But you need to call a doctor as soon as possible if you have black, tarry stool, which indicates blood in the digestive tract.

---

cially the lactose form of sugar found in many dairy products. Also keep an eye on starches, like those in breads and pastas, and soluble fiber found in many fruits and vegetables.

Chew, chew, chew. To avoid swallowing air, "eat more slowly," says Dr. Peura. "Chew well and with your mouth closed."

Give up milk. Avoid all milk products for a week to see how that affects your symptoms, says Naurang Agrawal, M.D., professor of medicine at the University of Connecticut School of Medicine in Farmington. "If the gas disappears, you are probably lactose intolerant."

Munch less fiber. Don't eat too much fiber, says Dr. Agrawal. "If you're sensitive to fiber, eating excessive amounts may lead to gas discomfort," he says. You might have to cut back on beans, whole grains, or nuts if you are too uncomfortable with the aftereffects.

Avoid sorbitol. A natural sugar also used in sugarless candies and gums, sorbitol tends to be poorly absorbed, says Dr. Phillips. "Avoid products made with sorbitol for a while and see if your symptoms improve."

Favor fennel. Drink a cup or two of fennel tea, says Brian Rees, M.D., medical director of Maharishi Ayur-Veda Medical Center in Pacific Palisades, California. "It's great for gas," he says.

Bet on Beano. This product, available at drugstores and many supermarkets, neutralizes raffinose, gas-producing sugar in beans, cabbage, brussel sprouts, and broccoli. Just add a few drops to gas-generating foods before you eat them.

Try a gas guzzler. Try an over-the-counter gas-reducing product that contains simethicone, says Marvin Schuster, M.D., former director of the division of digestive diseases at Johns Hopkins Bayview Medical Center in Baltimore. "These products help gas bubbles to coalesce, so you can pass the gas more easily," he says.

Genital Herpes

G enital herpes, or herpes simplex type 2, affects up to 20 percent of all sexually active people. This type of herpes typically begins with tingling or itching before the blisters appear.
After that, symptoms include painful open sores, a burning sensation
when urinating and, occasionally, muscle aches and fever.

The first outbreak is usually the most severe. After that, the
virus lurks inside nerve cells and flares in times of illness or stress and
during a woman's menstrual period. Flare-ups may also occur when
someone with herpes is exposed to other trigger factors such as heat
or sunlight.

Beating Pain to the Punch

The best way to control outbreaks of genital herpes is with the
prescription medications acyclovir (Zovirax) or famciclovir (Famvir).
If you take the medication as soon as the telltale tingling begins, you
may help to keep an outbreak in check, says Timothy Berger, M.D.,
associate clinical professor of dermatology at the University of California, San Francisco, School of Medicine. But if sores erupt, you'll
want to ease the pain. Here's what the experts recommend.

Apply cold compresses. Apply a piece of gauze or a washcloth soaked in cool water directly on the sores, suggests Clay J. Cockerell, M.D., associate professor of dermatology and pathology at the
University of Texas Southwestern Medical Center at Dallas. "Cool
compresses can help heal the lesions by drying them up," he says.

Soothe with salves. Dab your sores with a drying agent
such as calamine lotion, suggests Dudley Danoff, M.D., senior at-

When to See the Doctor

If you notice a blister that suddenly appears on your genitals or if you have sores that are causing severe pain, see your doctor, experts advise.

Also call your doctor if you have had an outbreak in the past and you feel tingling, itching, or tenderness at the site of a previous outbreak. "If you act quickly, you might be able to prevent an outbreak," says Timothy Berger, M.D., associate clinical professor of dermatology at the University of California, San Francisco, School of Medicine.

tending urologist at Cedars–Sinai Medical Center in Los Angeles and author of *Superpotency*.

Go for the silver. Apply colloidal silver directly to the sores, says Cynthia M. Watson, M.D., a family practitioner in private practice in Santa Monica, California. Available at health food stores, colloidal silver has antiviral and antibacterial action, she says. "When you use it, the lesions seem to dry up in a matter of days."

Try over-the-counter relief. For mild pain or discomfort, try a nonprescription nonsteroidal anti-inflammatory drug (NSAID) such as aspirin or ibuprofen, suggests Dr. Berger. Take the dosage recommended on the label.

Cutting Down on Outbreaks

The good news is that any subsequent outbreak of genital herpes will be milder than the first—and you may never develop a second one. To better your odds against repeated eruptions, follow these strategies.

Keep cool. Avoid sunbathing, saunas, and very hot baths and showers, especially if you start to feel the tingling sensation that precedes an outbreak, says Pamela Miller, a licensed acupuncturist at Balfour Chiropractic in Northridge, California. "Heat can be a trigger for recurrences," she says.

Defuse your triggers. Try to identify factors that seem to trigger your outbreaks and avoid them if possible, says Dr. Berger. "Some people develop an outbreak after they wear tight underwear, for example," he says.

Try to stay serene. Consider learning a stress-reduction technique such as progressive relaxation or meditation to reduce the severity and frequency of herpes, says Dr. Berger. "These techniques can help manage the disease by helping your immune system fight the virus more effectively," he says.

Get your antioxidants. Take a daily vitamin and mineral supplement that contains the antioxidants beta-carotene and vitamin C as well as zinc, suggests Dr. Watson. "These antioxidants can help heal the skin and fight infection," she says.

Look to lysine. Take 3 grams daily of this amino acid during an acute outbreak of genital herpes—then take 500 milligrams a day to help prevent recurrences, suggests Dr. Watson. "Lysine helps inhibit the duplication of the virus," she notes. You'll find lysine supplements in the vitamin section of drugstores or health food stores.

Consult with your doctor, however, before you take this supplement. In some people, "lysine can cause the liver to step up its production of cholesterol," says Melvyn Werbach, M.D., a physician in Los Angeles who specializes in nutritional medicine and the author of *Healing with Food.*

Gout

W hen your big toe makes direct contact with a bedpost, it hurts. When it's pinched by a too-tight shoe, it aches. But when it's attacked by gout . . . *yeowch!* Now you're talking serious pain.

The instigator of this agony is a chemical called uric acid. When your body produces too much of the acid or your kidneys can't get rid of it fast enough, the excess crystallizes in and around your joints—most likely in the joint of your big toe. This buildup produces swelling, tenderness, and pain so exquisite that just pulling a bedsheet over your foot is intolerable.

To make matters worse, gout offers no advance warning. One day your toe feels fine, the next day it feels as though it has been skewered with a hot poker. Flare-ups are infrequent at first but can become more regular over time. Left untreated, gout can actually damage the joint, producing stiffness and limiting movement.

Gout tends to run in families, often singling out overweight men who drink heavily or who eat lots of foods rich in purines. (When your body breaks down purines, the process produces uric acid.) Flare-ups can also be triggered by illness, injury, or crash dieting, among other factors.

This Little Piggy's in Pain

Doctors tend to favor medication as the first line of treatment for gout, according to Eric P. Gall, M.D., chairman of the department of medicine at Finch University of Health Sciences/Chicago Medical School. Certain prescription drugs can relieve your symptoms and defend against future attacks.

When to See the Doctor

You should consult your doctor any time you experience an acute attack of gout, says Arthur Grayzel, M.D., a rheumatologist and former spokesperson for the Arthritis Foundation. What qualifies as an acute attack? "The affected joint is usually red and warm to the touch, and you'll have a lot of pain," he says.

But there's a lot you can do on your own to help take the ouch out of gout, experts say. Here's what they recommend to get relief fast—and to reduce your risk of a recurrence.

Give it a break. During a bout with gout, rest the affected joint, says Arthur Grayzel, M.D., a rheumatologist and former spokesperson for the Arthritis Foundation. If it's your big toe that's hurting, "stay off your foot as much as possible and keep it elevated," he advises. Or walk with crutches.

Put it on ice. Apply ice to the affected joint for 20 minutes at a time, suggests Dr. Grayzel. Be sure to wrap the ice pack in a towel to protect your skin.

Take a "common-scents" approach. Aromatherapists recommend a cooling footbath to make a tender toe feel better. Their instructions: Add 10 drops each of the essential oils juniper and rosemary to 2 quarts of cold water, then immerse the affected foot for a good soak.

Hold the anchovies. Experts say that you can reduce your odds of a gout flare-up by monitoring your intake of purine-rich foods, such as anchovies, organ meats, broths, and gravies. These foods raise your body's level of uric acid—and too much uric acid is what leads to gout in the first place.

Ease up on imbibing. "Drinking too much alcohol raises the uric acid level in the blood," says Dr. Grayzel. You don't necessarily have to become a teetotaler, he notes. The key is moderation. Take notice of whether you routinely have gout attacks after you have been drinking alcohol.

Can the coffee. Coffee, tea, cola, and other foods and beverages that contain caffeine can negatively affect your body's uric acid level. "It's very individual, so pay attention," says Dr. Grayzel. "Sometimes an attack occurs if you exceed your usual intake of caffeine."

Skip the C. At times it seems that vitamin C is good for anything that ails you. But gout is an exception to the rule. "Avoid vitamin C supplements," advises Dr. Gall. "They can hamper the kidneys' ability to remove uric acid."

Help yourself to H$_2$O. Drinking large amounts of water helps flush away uric acid crystals, experts say. Try to drink at least 10 (8-ounce) glasses a day.

Pare pounds slowly. Because overweight has been linked to a high level of uric acid in the blood, slimming down may reduce your risk of a gout flare-up, Dr. Grayzel says. Just don't try to shed those pounds too fast. "Ironically, rapid weight loss may actually induce an attack," he notes.

Monitor your medication. Some blood pressure drugs can cause your uric acid level to rise, says Dr. Gall. What's more, some gout medicines don't work properly if they're taken with other drugs. So make sure that your doctor is aware of all the medications you're taking.

Wear sensible shoes. A minor injury caused by poorly fitting footwear can trigger a gout attack in your big toe, says Glenn Gastwirth, D.P.M., deputy executive director of the American Podiatric Medical Association. "Avoid shoes that are too tight or too narrow. You should be able to wiggle your toes freely."

Gum Pain

G um disease is serious business. Funny thing about it, though: Its symptoms are usually so subtle that you don't even realize the damage that is being done literally right under your nose.

Rather than feeling outright pain, you may experience a gnawing, itching, or burning sensation. You may notice a little bleeding when you brush or floss your teeth. It may be annoying, but it certainly doesn't seem like anything to worry about. Then during a routine checkup, your dental hygienist informs you that your gums have receded so much that one of your teeth has become wobbly.

The Dastardly Duo

The most common form of insidious gum disease is gingivitis. In fact, almost everyone develops some degree of gingivitis at some point in life, according to Jay W. Friedman, D.D.S., a dental consultant in Los Angeles and author of *Complete Guide to Dental Health*. The condition usually results from lapses in oral hygiene, which pave the way for the buildup of bacteria-laden plaque. This plaque buildup irritates the gums, causing them to become inflamed and to bleed. Eventually, the gums start receding, creating little pockets around the teeth where more plaque can make itself at home.

Left untreated, gingivitis can evolve into a more serious gum problem known as periodontitis. In periodontitis, the bacteria actually penetrate beneath the visible gum line and threaten the bone and tissues that support the teeth.

"With gingivitis or periodontitis, you may feel an itching sensation," says Kenneth M. Hargreaves, D.D.S., Ph.D., associate professor in the divisions of endodontics and pharmacology at the

When to See the Dentist

The earlier you catch gum disease, the more likely you will be able to stop it from progressing. Take any of the following symptoms as your cue to get to your dentist pronto: bleeding when you brush or floss, teeth that are loose or shaky, redness or tenderness in your gums, or blunting of the pointed triangles of gum tissue between your teeth.

"Don't delay getting to a dentist," cautions Kenneth M. Hargreaves, D.D.S., Ph.D., associate professor in the divisions of endodontics and pharmacology at the University of Minnesota Medical School in Minneapolis. "Gum disease will only get worse. If you ignore it, you can lose bone around your tooth, and the tooth can become loose and fall out. If the tooth is supporting dentures, you may not be able to wear your plate anymore because you will have lost the anchor that holds it in place. And if the tooth is part of a cemented-in bridge, you may lose the whole bridge."

Also keep an eye on any ulcers that develop on your gums. "Ulcers usually take 7 to 10 days to heal," says Lawrence Wolinsky, D.M.D., Ph.D., professor of oral biology at the University of California, Los Angeles, School of Dentistry. "If yours doesn't get better in that amount of time, see your dentist. It could be a sign of something more complex, such as an infection draining through the mouth or even a tumor."

University of Minnesota Medical School in Minneapolis. "But even that is uncommon. The great majority of patients with either condition have no change in sensation."

While periodontitis requires professional attention, gingivitis can be managed with proper hygiene—if it's detected soon enough. "Early diagnosis is very important," says Lawrence Wolinsky, D.M.D., Ph.D., professor of oral biology at the University of California, Los Angeles, School of Dentistry. "Gum disease is like high blood pressure. It doesn't always exhibit itself until it reaches an advanced stage. But if you catch it as gingivitis, it is easy to control and won't progress to periodontitis."

Just don't try to make the diagnosis yourself, experts caution. Let your dentist determine the exact nature of your condition.

Keep Your Gums in the Pink

What can you do when your dentist says that you have gum disease? Plenty. The following tips can help stop gingivitis in its tracks and restore gum health.

Keep it clean. Dentists emphasize that most cases of gum disease result from dental neglect: not brushing properly, not flossing, not having your teeth cleaned regularly. They also say that proper hygiene can often reverse gum deterioration before it gets out of hand.

What is meant by "proper hygiene"? Most experts say that you should brush three to five times a day, floss at least once—and preferably twice—a day, and see your dentist every six months.

Be gentle. While keeping your mouth clean is critical, you'll want to proceed gingerly when you have sore gums. "Patients with gum problems tend to get more vigorous with their brushing," says Dr. Wolinsky. "They think that they can brush the problem away. But they often end up inadvertently causing abrasions and ulcerations."

"Avoid aggressive brushing," agrees Robert Javer, D.M.D., a periodontist in private practice in the Boston area. "Make sure that you use a soft toothbrush. Plaque is a soft material and can be removed better with a soft brush than a hard one."

Make your own toothpaste. You can remove plaque gently and effectively with the following homemade preparation suggested by Howard S. Glazer, D.D.S., a dentist in Fort Lee, New Jersey, and past president of the Academy of General Dentistry: Combine one-quarter capful of 3 percent hydrogen peroxide (as opposed to the 10 percent hydrogen peroxide used to bleach hair) with enough baking soda to reach the consistency of sour cream. "This mixture causes an

Pain, Pain, Go Away

The good news is that your dentist says you don't have gum disease. The bad news is that your gums are still as sore as the dickens.

Infections, abrasions, and ulcers are just a few of the culprits behind painful gums. No matter what the cause, these tips will help ease your discomfort fast.

Try hydrogen peroxide. "If you have a minor infection, rinsing with hydrogen peroxide can provide temporary relief," says Jay W. Friedman, D.D.S., a dental consultant in Los Angeles and author of *Complete Guide to Dental Health.* "Just combine one part 3 percent hydrogen peroxide with one part water, swish the mixture around your mouth for about 30 seconds, then spit it out."

Soothe with salt water. To relieve swelling that's caused by infection, you can use a saltwater rinse on a temporary basis, says Robert Javer, D.M.D., a periodontist in private practice in the Boston area. His recommendation is to mix 1 teaspoon of salt in 1 cup of warm water. Hold the solution in the affected area of your mouth by leaning your head to that side for a while. Then spit out the solution. "You should go through a whole glass every 4 hours or so," he says. "If the swelling doesn't go down within 48 hours, see a dentist."

effervescent action," Dr. Glazer explains. "It gets into the pocket of the gum and cleans out some of the debris." After you brush your teeth, rinse with warm salt water, he adds.

Give up brushing—temporarily. If your gum tissue appears red or raw, Dr. Javer suggests that you forgo brushing that area for the time being so that it has a chance to heal. "Brushing will irritate the gum even more," he notes.

Instead of brushing, he says, dip a cotton swab in 3 percent hydrogen peroxide and dab the sore spot. "Hydrogen peroxide is a

Opt for baking soda. "You can mix 1 teaspoon of sodium bicarbonate (baking soda) in a glass of warm water and rinse your mouth with the solution," says Lawrence Wolinsky, D.M.D., Ph.D., professor of oral biology at the University of California, Los Angeles, School of Dentistry. Rinse after each brushing.

If you have heart disease or high blood pressure, be aware that many commercial mouth rinses contain high concentrations of sodium. "Don't swallow," Dr. Wolinsky cautions. "Just rinse and spit out. That way, not much sodium will be absorbed."

Find your salve-ation. For abrasions, Dr. Javer recommends an over-the-counter mouth-pain ointment called Zilactin. "It can be quite soothing," he says.

Consume carefully. If you have a sore or an ulcer on your gums, avoid eating anything that can irritate the tissue. "Stay away from spicy and acidic foods and drinks," says Dr. Wolinsky. This includes tomato juice and even colas. "They have pHs in the range of five, which is acidic," he notes.

What about orange juice? Dr. Wolinsky says that it's okay, provided you dilute it with water. "This reduces the acidic concentration, so the juice won't burn when you drink it," he explains.

cleansing agent," Dr. Javer explains. "If you use it for five to seven days, it will help clean the area and allow the gum to heal without toothbrush abrasion."

"You can brush the biting surface of the back teeth directly," he adds. "Just make sure that the brush doesn't touch the gum line."

Enlist a rinse. To treat gingivitis, Dr. Wolinsky recommends using a rinse with antiplaque properties. "It helps reduce the amount of plaque mass in your mouth at any one time," he explains.

Your best bet, he says, is a rinse that contains chlorhexidine

(Peridex). Since such products are available only by prescription, you should ask your dentist whether one would be right for you. "Some over-the-counter rinses (such as Viadent and Listerine) have been shown to be effective in preventing plaque buildup, but they don't work as well as those with chlorhexidine," Dr. Wolinsky adds.

Hit the spot with tea. If your gums are bleeding, tea can make it stop. "Just place a wet tea bag on the area that's bleeding," Dr. Javer says. "The tannic acid will help the blood clot."

Stock up on C. "Vitamin C is probably the only nutrient that is released in connective tissue," Dr. Glazer says. "It can be helpful in fighting periodontitis." Ask your dentist or doctor to recommend the proper dosage for you. Usually, it's somewhere between 1,000 and 2,500 milligrams a day.

Note: Taking more than 1,200 milligrams of vitamin C a day may cause diarrhea in some people.

Stop smoking. If the threat of lung cancer and heart disease hasn't persuaded you to can the cigs, then sore gums probably won't do the trick either. Just know that smoking not only aggravates gum disease, it can cause it in the first place. "There is such a thing as nicotine stomatitis," Dr. Glazer notes. "It's an inflammation of the soft tissue of the mouth that comes from nicotine irritation."

Avoid aspirin. Your friends mean well when they tell you to put aspirin on your sore gums. But don't listen to this old wives' tale. "Never put aspirin directly on your gums," warns Dr. Friedman. "Yes, it may provide some temporary relief. But aspirin is a highly caustic chemical, and it's irritating to the gum tissue. It could cause a fairly serious acid burn."

Hangover

Your stomach is bubbling like a hot tub. Your tongue feels as though you licked the lint trap of your dryer. And your head—oh, your poor, pounding head—will surely explode if you dare open your eyes.

You had one drink too many last night, and now your body is paying the piper for your overindulgence. Your doctor would say that you're suffering from alcohol withdrawal. You probably know it as a hangover.

All that booze you consumed has irritated your stomach and produced a skull-splitting headache by overdilating the blood vessels in your head. And because alcohol is a diuretic, it makes your thirst unquenchable and compounds your headache pain.

Help for the "Moaning After"

Only time will heal a hangover. You say that you can't wait? Well, chin up: Experts say that the following strategies can subdue your symptoms—and maybe even head off hangovers down the road.

Pick some fruit. Fructose, the natural sugar in fruit, enhances your body's ability to burn off alcohol, according to Seymour Diamond, M.D., director of the Diamond Headache Clinic in Chicago. He suggests nibbling on cherries, grapes, or apples—all of which are especially good sources of fructose. Or spread honey, another high-fructose food, on a piece of toast or some crackers.

Sip a sports drink. Being a diuretic, alcohol makes you urinate more frequently. That can lead to dehydration. "Sports drinks such as Gatorade can help replenish fluid and depleted minerals," says

When to See the Doctor

A hangover seldom requires medical treatment. But experts advise consulting your doctor if your headache lasts for more than a day or if nausea lingers for more than two days. You should also seek professional help if your hangovers become more frequent or severe or begin to interfere with your work, says John Brick, Ph.D., a biological psychologist and executive director of Intoxikon International, an organization in Yardley, Pennsylvania, that evaluates alcohol- and drug-related information for law-enforcement agencies.

John Brick, Ph.D., a biological psychologist and executive director of Intoxikon International, an organization in Yardley, Pennsylvania, that evaluates alcohol- and drug-related information for law-enforcement agencies.

Soothe your belly with bouillon. A cup of bouillon makes an ideal morning-after breakfast, Dr. Diamond says. It goes down easy on your grumbly stomach, and it helps replenish the salt, potassium, and other essential nutrients that alcohol siphons from your body.

Don't skip your java. If you always start your day with a cup of coffee, go ahead and have one, Dr. Brick urges. Doing without can make your hangover headache even worse.

Get your juices flowing. Because alcohol dehydrates, it can hinder the release of toxins such as lactic acid from your muscles, says Felice Dunas, Ph.D., a licensed acupuncturist and a doctor of clinical Chinese medicine in private practice in Topanga, California. This can leave you feeling stiff and crampy. "Take 10 to 15 minutes to stretch," Dr. Dunas advises. "It can improve your circulation and thus reduce the level of lactic acid."

Swallow a pill. Over-the-counter pain relievers remain a tried-and-true antidote to an alcohol-induced headache. Aspirin or ibuprofen is your best bet, Dr. Brick says—but don't take it until at least 4 hours after imbibing. Otherwise, the medication can further irritate an already angry stomach.

Pop C before you party. Vitamin C may help you bypass a hangover by helping your body get rid of alcohol faster. In a study at the University of South Florida College of Medicine in Tampa, 13 men took 2,000 milligrams of vitamin C an hour before drinking 5 ounces of whiskey. They also drank whiskey without taking vitamin C beforehand. In more than half the men, the level of alcohol in their blood decreased more rapidly when they took the vitamin C than when they didn't.

Note: Some people may experience diarrhea when taking more than 1,200 milligrams of vitamin C a day.

Pace yourself. Nurse your drink and sip a nonalcoholic beverage between drinks, Dr. Brick suggests. A tall glass of sparkling water with a twist of lime or a mix of cranberry juice and seltzer can be just as festive as a glass of wine or a mug of beer.

Skip salty snacks. Bypass nuts, chips, and other salt-laden munchies that make you thirsty, Dr. Brick advises. You may find that you don't need another drink after all.

Stick with high-protein fare. Dr. Diamond recommends noshing on foods that have lots of protein, such as cheese. They stay in your digestive system longer, so they help soak up alcohol, he explains. This reduces your risk of becoming intoxicated—and of waking up with a hangover.

Hit the water bottle, then hit the sack. After an evening of imbibing, drink as much water as you can before you go to bed, Dr. Brick advises. It helps protect against dehydration.

Headache

A nineteenth-century etching portrays headache pain as six gremlins simultaneously committing assorted torturous misdeeds against some poor soul's aching cranium. Judging by that image, it's safe to say that while a lot has changed over the past hundred years or so, headaches certainly haven't.

These days, some 45 million of us suffer from recurring headaches. And we spend almost $4 billion a year trying to get rid of them. One health expert has labeled them a universal plague.

Despite how common headaches are, everyone experiences them just a bit differently. Medical researchers have defined three general categories of headache pain.

- Tension headaches occur when the muscles in the head and neck contract and stay tense. The pain has been likened to putting your skull in a vise.
- Cluster headaches are characterized by searing pain on just one side of the head, usually around or behind the eye.
- Migraines produce throbbing pain that may be accompanied by vomiting, diarrhea, sweating, or chills. (For a more in-depth discussion of migraine, see page 170.)

Since any headache makes you feel miserable, distinguishing between the three categories may seem like splitting hairs. But experts say you should know which type you are prone to, especially if your pain is chronic. It enables you to manage your pain more effectively.

Rx for an Aching Head

As intense and disturbing as headache pain can be, it very seldom signals the onset of a life-threatening condition. That may not

When to See the Doctor

If you have chronic headaches, you should bring it to your doctor's attention, experts agree. Once your doctor has diagnosed the source of your pain, watch for significant changes in your symptoms, says Jerome Goldstein, M.D., assistant clinical professor of neurology at the University of California, San Francisco, School of Medicine and director of the San Francisco Headache Clinic. "See your doctor immediately if your headaches increase in frequency, duration, or severity or if they are accompanied by numbness, weakness on one side of your body, or difficulty with your speech, balance, or thought processes," he advises.

You should seek medical attention without delay if your headache is accompanied by a fever or a stiff neck, if it lasts for more than 24 hours, or if you have sustained a head injury.

be much comfort, though, when you're feeling as though the entire U.S. Olympic boxing team has been using your head for a punching bag. Here's what the experts say you should do to get relief fast—and to head off headache in the future.

Send the pain packing. Wrap a frozen gel pack in a towel and place it directly on the area that hurts, recommends Seymour Diamond, M.D., director of the Diamond Headache Clinic in Chicago and author of *The Hormone Headache*. Apply the pack for up to an hour, once or twice a day. You can purchase gel packs in drugstores and medical supply stores.

Feel the heat. Apply a heating pad to your neck and shoulders to relax tight neck and shoulder muscles and ease a tension headache, suggests Robert Kunkel, M.D., staff physician at the Headache Center of the Cleveland Clinic Foundation. Or take a hot shower, allowing the water to beat on your neck and shoulders and loosen the muscles.

Breathe better. Deep-breathing exercises can help put an end to headache pain, according to Dr. Diamond. Here is a simple one that he recommends: Lie on your back on a bed or the floor. Exhale completely, pulling in your abdominal muscles. Then slowly and gently inhale through your nose while expanding your abdomen. Imagine that you are breathing in a sense of ease, quiet energy, and well-being. Allow the breath to flow down to the bottom of your lungs. Your chest should expand slightly, but your shoulders should not rise.

When your lungs feel full, make a slow, smooth transition between inhaling and exhaling. Begin slowly exhaling through your mouth while contracting your abdominal muscles. Gently blow your breath away from you, through your mouth. Allow a sense of quiet to take over your body. Repeat the entire sequence a total of three times, Dr. Diamond says.

Put your finger on relief. Applying pressure to a point on your hand can help ease headache pain, according to Ira Klemons, D.D.S., Ph.D., director of the Center for Head and Facial Pain in South Amboy, New Jersey. To find the point, close up the thumb and index finger on one hand so that a crease forms between the two. You'll notice a small bump above the crease. Put the thumb of your opposite hand on the bump, then separate your thumb and index finger. If you push around a little bit, you'll find a point that's very tender when you have a headache. Firmly press on that point for about a minute, then switch hands. Repeat if the pain returns.

Head for your medicine chest. Over-the-counter pain relievers such as aspirin, ibuprofen, and acetaminophen are still the treatment of choice for many folks bothered by headaches, Dr. Diamond says. These medications work equally well, so which one you choose is really a matter of personal preference. "But you shouldn't be using painkillers on a daily or almost-daily basis," he cautions. "If you are, you should see your doctor."

Cool it on caffeine. One cup of coffee or another caffeinated beverage may help halt a headache. More than that can actually trigger a headache. "The more caffeine you consume, the more

---

If It's a Headache, It Must Be Saturday

Does it seem as though most of your headaches occur on weekends? It could be because you're upsetting your Monday-through-Friday routine, experts say. "If you go against your body's internal clock, certain metabolic processes can start too late or too early in the day and lead to a headache," explains R. Michael Gallagher, D.O., director of the University Headache Center at the University of Medicine and Dentistry of New Jersey School of Osteopathic Medicine in Stratford.

To keep your body's functions on schedule, you should try to get up at the same time every day—including Saturdays and Sundays. And while you're up, don't forget to have your morning coffee. "Many people get weekend headaches because they sleep in and miss their usual dose of caffeine," Dr. Gallagher notes.

likely you are to experience headaches," says Melvyn Werbach, M.D., a physician in Los Angeles who specializes in nutritional medicine and the author of *Healing with Food.*

If you need to cut down on caffeine, do so gradually, he advises. Otherwise, you might develop a caffeine-withdrawal headache. "It usually starts about 18 hours after you drink your last caffeinated beverage and peaks 3 to 6 hours later," he notes.

Learn to relax. "Prolonged stress can cause the muscles in your neck and shoulders to tighten, leading to a tension headache," says R. Michael Gallagher, D.O., director of the University Headache Center at the University of Medicine and Dentistry of New Jersey School of Osteopathic Medicine in Stratford. "When you feel those muscles tensing up, that's the time to slow down and, if you can, to remove yourself from the stressful situation."

In fact, you don't have to wait until you're tense to take action, Dr. Gallagher says: "Allow yourself some time every day for relaxation. Find a way to interrupt your stress, even if only for a half-hour."

Don't go hungry. "You're more prone to get headaches if you go for long periods of time without eating," Dr. Gallagher says. "The theory is that skipping meals causes changes in blood sugar, which in turn trigger a reaction in your body that sets you up for a headache."

Move it. Staying in one position for too long—whether you're hunched over your desk at work or curled up on the sofa watching television—can contribute to a headache, according to Dr. Kunkel. "Get up frequently and stretch your muscles," he urges.

Don't go undercover. Burying your head underneath a blanket while you sleep increases the level of carbon dioxide in your blood, Dr. Diamond notes. Because carbon dioxide constricts blood vessels, you might wake up with a headache.

Have no fear. Figuring out what causes your headaches and then staying away from those triggers is important, experts agree. But avoidance carried to an extreme can itself become a trigger, explains Mark Goulston, M.D., assistant clinical professor of psychiatry at the University of California, Los Angeles, UCLA School of Medicine and author of *Get Out of Your Own Way.* "It can make you tense, and the more tense you are, the easier it is to get a headache," he says. His advice: Try to distinguish real triggers from imagined ones and learn how to manage stressful situations rather than evading them.

Heartburn

You knew better. Still, you couldn't pass up the Fiesta Feast at your favorite Mexican restaurant. Now, after eating every last morsel of cheese-laden burrito and jalapeño-laced salsa, your gut has begun to protest in earnest. All that hot and spicy fare has ignited a four-alarm blaze right beneath your rib cage.

That fire-in-the-furnace feeling is the calling card of gastroesophageal reflux—in plain English, heartburn. Acid has backed up from your stomach into your esophagus, producing a burning, gnawing sensation that may spread from the middle of your chest to your throat and even to your face.

Experts don't yet know for sure what makes stomach acid head north in the first place. They do know that it has a lot to do with what and how you eat. Among the primary suspects: consuming meals that are too big, too heavy, or too fatty; drinking alcohol or smoking before or after a meal; and lying down immediately after a meal.

Putting Out the Fire Permanently

Of course, when heartburn strikes, you probably care less about what caused it than what can cure it. Traditionally, antacids have been the remedy of choice. But next time you feel the burn, try an over-the-counter medication called an acid inhibitor, suggests Scott Brazer, M.D., associate professor of medicine at Duke University Medical Center in Durham, North Carolina. Ask your doctor or pharmacist to recommend one or look for a brand name such as Tagamet HB. "Acid inhibitors are somewhat more effective than antacids and can actually prevent as well as treat heartburn," he says. They work by decreasing the amount of acid that is produced by the stomach.

When to See the Doctor

Heartburn may be a symptom of another, more serious health problem. You should seek medical attention without delay if you notice that the pain occurs primarily with exertion, is moving down your left arm, or is accompanied by shortness of breath or difficulty swallowing, advises Scott Brazer, M.D., associate professor of medicine at Duke University Medical Center in Durham, North Carolina. You should also see your doctor if your heartburn doesn't go away within three weeks, despite treatment with home remedies, or if it awakens you from your sleep. It may be a sign that your heart muscle is not getting enough oxygen.

Don't rely on an over-the-counter drug indefinitely. If heartburn persists for more than three weeks, see your doctor as soon as possible. To head off future bouts of heartburn, heed the following advice.

Don't eat the whole thing. "A large, heavy meal distends the stomach, which in turn spreads the esophageal muscle," explains Melvyn Werbach, M.D., a physician in Los Angeles who specializes in nutritional medicine and the author of *Healing with Food*. This allows the contents of your stomach to creep back up into your esophagus, causing heartburn.

Avoid aggravating foods. Try not to consume foods and beverages that trigger heartburn, says Dr. Werbach. These include fatty and spicy dishes, chocolate, alcohol, coffee, tea, milk, orange juice, and tomato juice.

Create a relaxing repast. Emotional distress increases the secretion of stomach acid, Dr. Werbach explains. "It's important to maintain a sense of calm, especially during and after meals."

Stay hydrated. Drink plenty of water, especially after a meal, says Dr. Werbach. "Water soothes the irritated lining of the esophagus by flushing the mixture of food and acid back into the stomach," he notes.

Give up pre-sleep treats. Dr. Brazer recommends that you don't eat anything within 3 hours of your bedtime. And don't lie down for a snooze after dinner. The reason is that acid reflux is more likely to occur when you're lying down than when you're sitting or standing. "When you're upright, gravity tends to clear the esophagus of acid," he says. Also, while you're awake, you're making saliva and swallowing it, which helps wash acid from the esophagus.

Hold your head high. If your heartburn is severe, keep your head elevated while you're in bed, advises Dr. Brazer. "Get gravity to work in your favor," he says. You can use a few pillows or, even better, put wooden blocks under the bedposts at the head of your bed.

Mind your medication. Some prescription drugs can contribute to heartburn, says David Peura, M.D., associate professor of medicine at the University of Virginia Health Sciences Center in Charlottesville. Nonsteroidal anti-inflammatory drugs (NSAIDs), for example, damage the lining of the stomach, so you may need to coat your stomach before taking one of these drugs. "If you are taking medication for a chronic condition and are experiencing heartburn, consult your doctor," he suggests.

Heel Pain

Time may heal all wounds. But it takes much more than time to heal a heel. "Perhaps the biggest mistake that people make is thinking that heel pain is eventually going to go away on its own," explains Rock Positano, D.P.M., co-director of the Foot and Ankle Orthopedic Institute at the Hospital for Special Surgery in New York City. "Sometimes they wait as long as six months before deciding that they need to see a doctor. But unlike other parts of the body, the foot is weight bearing, so when the heel is injured, the inflammation persists."

Like the rest of your foot, your heel is designed for shock absorption. The cushiony outer pad and the underlying bone—the largest of the 26 bones in your foot—can withstand the tremendous impact that occurs when you walk or run.

But your heel bone has an ample blood supply, which makes it softer and spongier than other bones, Dr. Positano explains. It has an ample nerve supply, too.

"Many nerves run down the leg through the heel and on to other parts of the foot," he says. "Both of these traits make the heel very susceptible to injury."

Your heel can hurt for any number of reasons. Perhaps the most common is inflammation or tearing of the plantar fascia, a band of fibrous connective tissue that runs along the bottom of the foot from the heel bone across the arch to the toes. This condition, known as plantar fasciitis, can cause pain that radiates from the heel to other parts of the foot.

Heel pain can also be caused by everything from poorly fitting shoes to biomechanical problems when you walk or run. Conditions such as tendinitis and rheumatoid arthritis can aggravate the heel as well.

Heel-Friendly Footwear

People who have heel pain must be extra careful in their selection of shoes. While the right pair can give your heel much-needed support, the wrong pair can make your pain even worse.

When you're shopping for shoes, heed this advice from the experts.

Fit your foot right. It may be the style of a shoe that catches your eye, but it's the sole that really counts. Turn the shoe over and run a line down the sole from the middle of the heel to the toes. "You should have about a 50-50 distribution on the left and right sides of the line at the ball of the foot," notes Phyllis Ragley, D.P.M., a podiatrist in Lawrence, Kansas, and president of the American Academy of Podiatric Sportsmedicine. "An uneven distribution takes away some support in the arch and strains the plantar fascia."

Look for other qualities. "A shoe should have ample support, a small heel—¼ to ½ inch in thickness—and a flexible sole," Dr. Ragley adds. "The last thing you want is a stiff shoe."

Replace them often. A shoe that is worn out won't give your heel the support and shock absorption it needs, says Pamela Colman, D.P.M., director of health affairs for the American Podiatric Medical Association. "You should evaluate a shoe as you would a tire," she says. "If the tread goes down or wears out on one side, it's time for a new pair."

Nursing a Hurting Heel

Because the heel is so vulnerable to such an assortment of problems, experts suggest that you have any pain evaluated by your doctor. That way, you can be certain of its cause and receive proper treatment.

Once your pain has been diagnosed, a healthy dose of pa-

When to See the Doctor

It's a good idea to have any heel pain checked out by your doctor, experts say. That way your doctor can rule out more serious conditions and prescribe an appropriate course of treatment.

A visit to the doctor is especially called for if you experience any of the following, says Phyllis Ragley, D.P.M., a podiatrist in Lawrence, Kansas, and president of the American Academy of Podiatric Sportsmedicine.

- Persistent pain
- Swelling—especially if you can't discern the anklebone from the back of the heel
- Discoloration
- Difficulty standing on the heel
- Any significant change in feeling or function
- Tenderness when you squeeze the heel from the sides

tience is in order: A wounded heel can take weeks or even months to heal. In the meantime, the following tips can help speed your recovery.

Run hot and cold. Use cold treatments for the first 48 hours after heel pain starts, advises Pamela Colman, D.P.M., director of health affairs for the American Podiatric Medical Association. Experts suggest simply massaging your heel with an ice cube for 5 to 7 minutes, until the area becomes numb. You can do this three to four times a day or as needed.

"Then after 48 hours, begin alternating between cold and hot treatments," Dr. Colman says. "Apply an ice pack for 15 minutes, wait for 15 minutes, then apply a moist heating pad for 15 minutes." Do this once a day.

Mend with medicine. "A nonsteroidal anti-inflammatory drug (NSAID) such as ibuprofen can help reduce any inflammation," Dr. Colman says. Ask your doctor or pharmacist to recommend one.

Cushion your heel. "A heel cushion provides support and protection, which can relieve pain and swelling," Dr. Colman says. This device is available in drugstores, both over the counter and by prescription. There are many kinds, too, from doughnut-shaped to cup-shaped. Which type of cushion you should use depends on the nature of your condition as well as other factors, she says. For this reason, you may want to talk to your doctor or pharmacist before purchasing one.

Go a little higher. If you have plantar fasciitis, a heel-raiser may provide some relief, Dr. Positano says. This device, which is sold over the counter in drugstores, inserts in your shoe and raises your heel by ⅛ to ¼ inch. "This takes some of the pressure off the point where the plantar fascia inserts into the heel," he explains. "This means the plantar fascia has to work less."

Opt for orthotics. Orthotics are custom-fitted shoe inserts that can ease your heel pain and perhaps fix the problem that is causing it. "Some heel problems have biomechanical origins," Dr. Positano explains. "Because the foot is not functioning properly, certain parts of it—such as the heel—have to work harder, which causes them to hurt. A prescription orthotic, given by a doctor, can correct the condition."

Loosen up. "A tight heel cord can cause pain in the heel and the arch," says Glenn Gastwirth, D.P.M., deputy executive director of the American Podiatric Medical Association. "Stretching it can relieve a lot of pain and sometimes even make other treatment unnecessary."

He suggests this exercise: Stand at arm's length from a wall. Place your palms on the wall, shoulder-width apart. Step back with your right foot, bending your left knee slightly. Lean toward the wall and drop your right heel to the ground. You will feel some pull or tightness in the back of your right calf. If it's too uncomfortable, move closer to the wall, bringing your right foot in a little bit. Hold the stretch for a count of 10, then switch legs. Repeat the exercise 5 to 10 times per leg.

As you do this exercise, be sure not to bounce on your heel. "You want a gradual, gentle stretch," Dr. Gastwirth says. "Tugging or sudden pulling can injure the tissue."

Hemorrhoids

L ots of things—bills, bosses, parking tickets—are a pain in the butt. But having a hemorrhoid tops the list. A hemorrhoid is really just a varicose vein that sprouts "where the sun don't shine." The colloquial name, piles, means more than one hemorrhoid.

Are you likely to get them? Well, people who have chronic constipation or who habitually strain to move their bowels are susceptible. So are pregnant women, as the expanding uterus compresses the veins and obstructs the return of blood from the rectum. But they're so common that you may not be able to identify a specific cause.

Sometimes you don't even know that you have hemorrhoids. But in many cases, they refuse to be ignored, causing symptoms such as itching, bleeding, and pain.

Turning "Ouch" to "Ah"

If you suspect that you have hemorrhoids, see your doctor. If you know that you have them, try these pain-relief tips.

Sit in a sitz bath. Sit in a tub filled with 6 to 8 inches of warm water for 10 minutes, three times a day, suggests Max M. Ali, M.D., director of Hemorrhoid Clinics of America in Oak Park, Michigan. "Add 1 cup of Epsom salts if you wish. It can help reduce the swelling and can be quite soothing."

Reach for a tube of relief. For temporary relief, apply a nonprescription hemorrhoid preparation (such as Preparation H), suggests Dr. Ali. "Both ointments and suppositories are quite effective," he says. No need to spend a bundle on these salves, however. "Most of them are based on a similar formula," says Dr. Ali, so you can get

When to See the Doctor

If you develop bleeding from your rectum or experience a change in your bowel habits—or if the pain is severe—see your doctor, says Max M. Ali, M.D., director of Hemorrhoid Clinics of America in Oak Park, Michigan.

the generic brand rather than name-brand ointment. "You can also use plain old nonmedicated petroleum jelly," he adds.

Try a pain-relieving pad. Apply a hemorrhoid ointment or cream directly to the hemorrhoid, then cover the area with a sanitary napkin that has been soaked in Epsom salts, suggests Dr. Ali. (To make sure that the pad stays in place, attach it to your underwear.) "Or try the medicated pads (such as Tucks) for hemorrhoids—they serve the same purpose," he says.

Wipe gingerly. Wipe with moistened toilet paper, which is less abrasive, suggests John A. Flatley, M.D., retired clinical instructor of surgery at the University of Missouri—Kansas City School of Medicine. And wipe gently: "Rough toilet hygiene can irritate a hemorrhoid," he says. Also, avoid using scented or colored toilet paper, which contains chemicals that may irritate hemorrhoids.

Get off the pot. Don't spend too long on the toilet, advises Dr. Flatley. "It encourages the formation of hemorrhoids."

Do some serious guzzling. The harder your stool, the harder you have to push, which can aggravate hemorrhoids. "Water is cheaper than a stool softener, and it's just as effective," says Dr. Flatley. He suggests that you should try to drink at least eight 8-ounce glasses of water a day.

But if water doesn't help, try a mild, over-the-counter stool softener, adds Dr. Ali. If you are salt sensitive and you have high blood pressure, just make sure that the softener you choose doesn't contain sodium.

Eat more fiber. To keep your stool soft, consume a high-fiber diet, especially during a flare-up, says Dr. Ali. "Eat more fresh fruits and vegetables and less red meat and cheese."

Exercise—but not too hard. You should avoid activities that put a strain on hemorrhoids such as lifting weights or cycling, advises Dr. Ali. He recommends swimming. You can resume your usual exercise routine once the flare-up is over. "Regular exercise can help prevent hemorrhoids by helping to regulate your bowel movements," he says.

Hip Pain

Your hips sure come in handy at times. They're perfectly located for supporting extra-heavy grocery bags or for giving an open car door a shove when your hands are full. But they were never intended as your body's built-in valet. If anything, they are more a combination of bodyguard and chauffeur. They provide indispensable protection for your vital organs and give your legs the range of motion they need to carry you from one place to another.

In fact, it's when you are on the move that your hips are at greatest risk for injury. A bad fall or a blow to the knee can cause the hip joint to dislocate—in other words, the hipbone no longer connects to the thighbone. The hip joint is also a prime candidate for arthritis. And the muscles and tendons that support the hips can become strained and inflamed from overuse.

To complicate matters, most of your body's large muscle groups span your hips. That means the pain you feel may come not from the hip joints but from the spine, lower back, buttocks, or some other location.

Hip, Hip, Hooray! Relief at Last

Because hip pain has so many potential causes, your best bet is to have it evaluated by your doctor, experts say. While you're waiting for your appointment, or if your doctor has already ruled out a more serious problem, the following strategies can help you nurse your hip back to health.

Go polar. Ice is the first line of defense against hip pain, says John Cianca, M.D., assistant professor of physical medicine and rehabilitation at Baylor College of Medicine in Houston. His suggestion is

Fending Off Fractures

A mong people over age 65, one of the most common causes of hip pain is fracture. Your risk of sustaining this type of injury increases over time, as you continue to lose bone mass. But the following strategies—based on guidelines from the American Academy of Orthopedic Surgeons—will help keep your hips healthy and strong, says William J. Robb III, M.D., senior attending orthopedic surgeon at Evanston and Glenbrook Hospitals in Evanston, Illinois.

Supplement your diet. Make sure that you're getting enough calcium and vitamin D. The amount of calcium you need every day depends on your age and gender.

- Women ages 25 to 50: 1,000 milligrams
- Women at menopause (ages 51 to 65) who are taking estrogen: 1,000 milligrams
- Women at menopause (ages 51 to 65) who are not taking estrogen: 1,500 milligrams
- Men ages 25 to 65: 1,000 milligrams
- Men and women over age 65: 1,500 milligrams

As for vitamin D, which your body needs to process calcium, aim for 400 international units per day.

Exercise regularly. Exercise is important for maintaining strong bones. It also improves your balance and reflexes, making you less likely to fall.

Break bad habits. Smoking and excessive alcohol consumption both increase your risk of fracture and impede healing.

Create a fall-safe environment. Make sure that you have secure rugs, good lighting throughout your home, sturdy handrails on stairways, nonskid strips and grab bars in bathtubs, and slip-resistant carpeting on the bathroom floor.

Get regular checkups. Your doctor should periodically evaluate the status of your bone mass, especially if you have a family history of osteoporosis.

to "crush some ice and place it in a resealable storage bag, so it has a greater surface area. Lay a thin towel over your hip, then apply the ice at the site of pain for 15 minutes."

If your pain is acute—caused by an injury, for example—you may need to reapply the ice as often as once every hour, Dr. Cianca says. But for chronic pain such as arthritis, once or twice a day may be enough.

Change the temperature. After 48 hours of cold treatment, start using heat instead, says Ramon Jimenez, M.D., chief of staff at O'Connor Hospital in San Jose, California, and president of the California Orthopedic Association. A heating pad on a low to medium setting will do. "But don't fall asleep on it," he warns.

You can also try soaking in a hot tub if you have access to one. "Keep the water in the 90°F range," Dr. Jimenez advises. "Ideally, the water temperature shouldn't exceed your body temperature."

Take a tablet. An over-the-counter pain reliever such as ibuprofen or acetaminophen can help a hurting hip, Dr. Jimenez says.

"But if the dosage recommended on the label doesn't do the trick, alert your doctor," Dr. Cianca adds. "Something more serious may be going on."

Be reasonable. Don't place too many demands on an aching hip, Dr. Jimenez cautions. In general, he says, stay away from any activity that aggravates your pain. You may have to drive to work instead of walking or take the elevator instead of bounding up three flights of stairs—at least for the time being.

Get some support. "If you can't walk without limping, then use crutches or a cane," advises William S. Case, president of Case Physical Therapy in Houston. When you try to avoid bearing weight on your sore hip, you can easily strain muscles and tendons in other areas.

If you opt for a cane, Dr. Jimenez reminds you to use proper technique: Carry the cane in the hand opposite the injured hip. Move it forward at the same time you step out with the injured hip, so you're bearing weight on both the good hip and the cane. Then step out with your "good" hip.

When to See the Doctor

In general, any pain in the hip region calls for a thorough examination by a physician, experts say. You want to be sure that no serious problem is causing your discomfort.

The following symptoms are particular cause for concern and should receive immediate medical attention, adds Thomas Rizzo, Jr., M.D., a physiatrist in the department of physical medicine and rehabilitation at the Mayo Clinic in Jacksonville, Florida.

- The pain persists after a couple of weeks, despite self-care that includes ice treatments and over-the-counter pain relievers.
- The pain shoots down your leg from the buttock area.
- The pain occurs while you lie in bed at night.
- You can't bear weight on the hip.

Walk in water. To keep your hip limber while you recover, head to your nearest pool for an aquatic workout, Dr. Jimenez suggests. "Water takes the weight off your hip and allows you to do more without pain than you could on dry land," he explains.

Flex some muscle. Stretching exercises can help relax the muscles in the hip region and improve flexibility, Dr. Cianca says. This is great not only for rehabilitating a sore hip but also for protecting against future problems.

Dr. Cianca recommends doing the following sequence once a day. Hold each position without bouncing and stretch only to the limit of comfort, he says. If you start to feel pain, stop.

1. Lie on your back on the floor. Place your right ankle over your left knee, making a figure 4 with your legs. Then raise your left leg, keeping it straight. Grasp it behind the thigh with your hands and pull it toward your chest. You will feel a stretch in your right buttock. Hold for 10 to 15 seconds, then switch legs.

2. Sit on the floor with your legs outstretched. Bend your right leg and cross it over your left leg. Your right foot should be flat on the ground on the outside of your left knee. Twist slightly so that you can press your left elbow against the outside of your right knee, pulling the knee toward you. Hold for 10 to 15 seconds, then switch legs.
3. Stand facing a waist-high table. Rest the lower part of your right leg on the table so that your right hip is flexed and your right leg is perpendicular to your body. Bend your whole body forward over your right leg. Hold for 10 to 15 seconds, then switch legs.

Strike a pose. Yoga can also enhance hip flexibility, says Arthur H. Brownstein, M.D., a physician in Princeville, Hawaii, and clinical instructor of medicine at the University of Hawaii School of Medicine in Manoa. He recommends this simple pose: Sit on the floor and place the soles of your feet together. Pull your feet in, as close to the groin as comfortable. Then let gravity pull your knees toward the floor. If this position is uncomfortable at first, he suggests modifying it slightly by bending only one leg at a time and keeping the other leg extended. Hold the pose for 15 seconds. Repeat three times.

Be patient. It's going to take a while for your hip to heal, especially if you have injured a muscle. "If you pull a hamstring muscle (located in the back of either thigh), it can take 6 to 10 weeks to get better," Dr. Jimenez notes.

Ready, set . . . slow. Once you have recovered enough to bear weight on your hip, make a gradual return to your usual routine. "Give yourself time," advises Phillip A. Bauman, M.D., clinical instructor in orthopedic surgery at the Columbia University College of Physicians and Surgeons and associate attending physician of orthopedic surgery at St. Luke's/Roosevelt Hospital Center, both in New York City. "Don't fall into the trap of doing too much too soon."

Ingrown Toenail

It seems the nail on your big toe has a very bad sense of direction. Instead of growing out straight, like a good nail should, it has taken a wrong turn into your skin. And boy oh boy, does it hurt. Just a slow walk to the corner mailbox can make your toe throb as if you dropped a bowling ball on it.

Podiatrists say that ingrown toenails are by far the most common nail problem. They usually affect the big toe, although every toe is vulnerable. They occur for any number of reasons: Too-tight shoes, fungal infection, injury, and constant pressure on the feet can all cause a toenail to dig into surrounding skin. But more often than not, an ingrown toenail is self-inflicted—the result of an overzealous pedicure.

Heal, Toe, Heal

An errant toenail usually inflicts enough pain that you'll attend to it pronto. But if you're inclined to just grin and bear it, you may want to reconsider. Left untreated, an ingrown nail can lead to inflammation or infection. Here's what you can do to make sure your nails toe the line.

Don't try to fix it. Home repairs can make an ingrown toenail even worse, cautions David C. Novicki, D.P.M., president of the American College of Foot and Ankle Surgeons. "People start excavating along the edge of the nail, and as they poke and prod, they nip the skin," he explains. "When that happens, it opens the door to a bad infection."

Dr. Novicki's warning is especially important if you have diabetes or a circulatory problem. "The risk is even greater," he notes.

Nailing Down Toenail Pain

Ingrown nails may be the most common cause of toenail pain. But other problems can plague the tender tips of your tootsies.

Because of their location, your toenails are especially vulnerable to injury—like when an oblivious shopper rolls a grocery cart over your foot, or a hammer slips out of your hand and takes dead aim at your big toe. Here are some other common causes of toenail pain.

Onycholysis. All or part of the nail becomes separated from the nail bed. This condition is especially common among ballet dancers, who exert a lot of pressure on the tips of their toes.

Paronychia. The skin around the nail becomes inflamed, most often as the result of a poorly fitting shoe.

Subungual hematoma. A hemorrhage underneath the nail, this is caused by a shearing or crushing injury.

These are serious conditions that require a doctor's examination and care, experts say. This is especially important if you have diabetes or a circulatory problem, adds Glenn Gastwirth, D.P.M., deputy executive director of the American Podiatric Medical Association.

"People with diabetes, for example, have decreased sensation in their feet. They might injure themselves without even realizing it."

Take a dip. Soaking your foot in warm water will soften the skin around the nail and reduce inflammation, says Rock Positano, D.P.M., co-director of the Foot and Ankle Orthopedic Institute at the Hospital for Special Surgery in New York City. For added therapeutic benefit, he suggests using an over-the-counter antibacterial solution such as Domeboro. Finish your soak by gently drying your foot, then applying an antibacterial ointment to the affected area, he says.

Pop a pill. An over-the-counter pain reliever can help ease inflammation, experts say. "I prefer the nonsteroidal kind," says Carol

---

When to See the Doctor

While an ingrown toenail is mighty painful, it usually doesn't require a doctor's attention. "But if you have any redness, swelling, or discharge in the area, it should be managed professionally," says Glenn Gastwirth, D.P.M., deputy executive director of the American Podiatric Medical Association.

If you have diabetes or a circulatory problem, do not try to treat an ingrown nail on your own, Dr. Gastwirth adds. These conditions can lead to diminished sensation in your feet. Should the ingrown nail become infected, you may not feel the physical symptoms, he explains.

Frey, M.D., a foot and ankle surgeon at the Orthopedic Hospital in Los Angeles. "There are many on the market—ibuprofen and naproxen (Aleve), for example. I usually recommend taking them for two weeks straight, then as needed. Just follow the directions on the label for the correct dosage."

Count on cotton. "You can get some relief by placing a small piece of cotton between the nail and the skin," says Dr. Novicki. But he cautions against being overzealous with this remedy. "People use toothpicks and other objects, and they do too much shoving and probing," he notes. "They can end up making the problem worse."

Opt for oil. "Rub baby oil or olive oil on the side of the nail," says Phyllis Ragley, D.P.M., a podiatrist in Lawrence, Kansas, and president of the American Academy of Podiatric Sportsmedicine. "It keeps the skin soft, so there is less pressure and discomfort. Also, the skin can more easily accommodate the nail."

Give it some room. If your ingrown nail is painful and swollen, don't confine it in tight-fitting shoes. "Wear an open-toed slipper or a sandal," Dr. Ragley suggests. "Or cut a hole in the toe box of an old shoe. The idea is to keep pressure off your toe."

Don't cut corners. Once your ingrown toenail has healed, you can prevent a recurrence by learning proper nail-trimming technique. Experts recommend using toenail clippers—not ordinary scissors—for your pedicure. "In general, always clip the nail straight across," says Glenn Gastwirth, D.P.M., deputy executive director of the American Podiatric Medical Association. "Don't cut too close. The nail should extend over the top ridge of flesh so that it has room to grow. And don't go fishing down the sides to try to extract a portion of the nail."

Buy spacious shoes. Tight-fitting shoes can cause a toenail to bury into your skin. So you want to make sure that your footwear has a lot of room up front. "You should be able to freely wiggle all of your toes," Dr. Frey advises. "There should be a half-inch between the end of your longest toe and the end of the toe box of the shoe."

"The toe box should be the right height, too, so that the tops of your toes don't rub against the shoe," Dr. Gastwirth adds. (For more tips on finding a shoe that's a good fit, see "Shoe-Shopping Savvy" on page 102.)

Intercourse Pain

S udden, intense pain has brought an abrupt end to your romantic interlude. Your partner is baffled and hurt. You're embarrassed and anxious. And you're both left to wonder: What could possibly cause this most exquisite of life's pleasures to become so indescribably excruciating?

It's a question that confronts many women—far more women than men. And it's not easy to answer. Because painful intercourse could have physical or psychological roots, you must look at your symptoms honestly before you can treat them effectively.

The physical causes of intercourse pain fall into two general categories, according to Emanuel Fliegelman, D.O., professor emeritus of obstetrics and gynecology and director of the human sexuality program at the Philadelphia College of Osteopathic Medicine. If it hurts when the penis is inserted, the vaginal opening is probably inflamed, too dry, or too narrow. If the pain occurs after insertion, it could indicate a bladder or pelvic infection.

For some women, though, intercourse pain stems not from a physical problem but from emotional distress. They may fear sexual contact or harbor deep-seated anger toward their partners.

No matter what its cause, even a single episode of painful intercourse can evolve into a vicious circle. You expect sex to hurt, which makes you tense. And if it already hurts, the additional tension can intensify your pain.

Take the Pain out of Passion

While there is plenty that you can do to put an end to intercourse pain, the one thing you should not do is ignore it. "In general,

When to See the Doctor

If intercourse is often painful, you should discuss it with your doctor, experts say. This is especially important when:
- Your pain is accompanied by a low-grade fever.
- You have an unusual amount of vaginal discharge.
- Your vaginal discharge has an unusual color or odor.
- Your pain persists for some time after intercourse.

If your doctor can't find a physical cause for your pain, you may want to consider counseling, says Hyla Cass, M.D., assistant clinical professor of psychiatry at the University of California, Los Angeles, UCLA School of Medicine. You may need help in dealing with some underlying emotional issue—anything from a marital rift to past abuse.

women don't feel comfortable talking about it," notes Donald DeWitt, M.D., clinical professor of family medicine at East Carolina University School of Medicine in Greenville, North Carolina. "They'd rather suffer in silence than open up, even to their partners." Unfortunately, this could have serious consequences, especially if your pain is produced by a condition such as endometriosis (which is an overgrowth of the tissue that lines the uterus).

If you're reluctant to take action, look at it this way: The sooner you pinpoint the source of your discomfort, the sooner you can resume a healthy physical relationship with your partner. So if you find intercourse consistently painful, see your doctor. In the meantime, here is what the experts recommend for relief.

Maximize moisture. If your pain results from vaginal dryness, experts recommend using a lubricating product (such as K-Y Jelly or Replens). But steer clear of petroleum jelly, Dr. Fliegelman cautions: "It's too sticky and gooey."

Ease the way with vitamin E. Applying vitamin E to the vagina can help heal dry, irritated tissue, according to Cynthia M.

When He Has Pain

Women experience intercourse pain far more frequently than men do. But that doesn't mean that men are immune. The skin of the penis can get irritated from too much friction within the vagina. The urethra (the tube that carries urine from the bladder) or prostate can become inflamed, making ejaculation painful. Or the head of the penis can feel sore, the result of infection with the human papillomavirus.

Perhaps the most serious intercourse-related condition that affects men is priapism—basically, an erection that won't let up. Don't think for a minute that this is a good thing: Priapism hurts like crazy, and experts warn that it can lead to permanent problems if it's left untreated.

Any one of these conditions will probably cause you enough discomfort to send you to your doctor—and that's exactly what you should do, experts say. (For more information about treating penile pain, see the chapter on page 190.)

Watson, M.D., a family practitioner in private practice in Santa Monica, California, and author of *Love Potions*. She suggests either pricking a vitamin E capsule and squeezing out the oil or using the vitamin in liquid form (it's available in health food stores and drugstores). Repeat the treatment several times a week.

Note: Vitamin E is not a lubricant and should not be used during intercourse, Dr. Watson advises.

Put the squeeze on pain. Consciously working the pubococcygeal (PC) muscle, located at the bottom of the pelvis between the anus and the genitals, can teach you to relax the muscle during intercourse, says Felice Dunas, Ph.D., a licensed acupuncturist and a doctor of clinical Chinese medicine in private practice in Topanga, California, and author of *Passion Play*. This helps make penetration less painful.

"You hold in urine by contracting the PC muscle," Dr. Dunas

says. "So practice squeezing the muscle three times whenever you urinate. You should squeeze hard enough to stop the flow of urine." She also suggests exercising the muscle before you go to sleep: Squeeze it as tight as you can, hold for a count of 5 to 10, then relax. Repeat a total of three times.

Get a new prescription. Taking low-dose birth control pills for a long period of time may cause the vaginal tissue to become thinner, setting the stage for intercourse pain, says David Redwine, M.D., director of the Endometriosis Institute in Bend, Oregon. You may want to talk to your doctor about changing your prescription, he suggests.

Wait until you're ready. "A woman should be highly stimulated before penetration occurs," according to Dr. Dunas. This has two benefits, she says: It ensures that the vagina is sufficiently lubricated, and it lengthens the vagina to accommodate deep thrusting.

Explore your options. If one sexual position seems to cause you pain, then you and your partner should experiment to find something more comfortable. For example, if you have a problem with deep penetration, Dr. Dunas suggests trying a position that lengthens the vagina somewhat. Lying on your back with your legs straight out rather than up may help, she says.

Be honest. Talking about a sexual problem with your partner is seldom easy, Dr. Fliegelman says. But if you let your partner know what hurts, you open the door to a frank and honest discussion—and the two of you may come up with a solution together.

Irritable Bowel Syndrome

A surly spouse may frustrate you. A boorish boss may aggravate you. But no matter how hard they try, neither one could ever match the misery caused by a ticked-off bowel.

Irritable bowel syndrome (IBS)—also known as colitis or spastic colon—is a chronic intestinal disorder characterized by abdominal pain and cramps, constipation, and diarrhea. Flare-ups can usually be traced to something you've eaten. Among the most common triggers are milk and dairy products, spicy foods, fatty foods, and gas-producing foods such as beans, broccoli, cabbage, and cauliflower.

If you're a woman, you may also experience symptoms as a result of hormonal fluctuations that occur during the menstrual cycle. This may explain why IBS affects three times as many women as men.

The frequency and intensity of flare-ups can vary greatly from one person to the next. Some folks barely notice their symptoms, while others must cope with crushing pain as well as urgent trips to the bathroom. While experts can't yet explain the disparity, they suggest that emotional stress plays a key role in increasing the severity of IBS.

Calming a Grumbly Gut

While IBS is a chronic condition, most people can successfully minimize flare-ups just by watching what they eat and managing the stress in their lives. If you want to lessen your digestive distress, give these strategies a try.

Take notes. Keeping a food diary can help you detect the dietary sources of your IBS flare-ups, says Marvin Schuster, M.D.,

When to See the Doctor

Seek medical attention right away if you develop extreme abdominal pain or have diarrhea for more than a day or two. You should also alert your doctor if you experience rectal bleeding, advises Naurang Agrawal, M.D., professor of medicine at the University of Connecticut School of Medicine in Farmington.

former director of the division of digestive diseases at Johns Hopkins Bayview Medical Center in Baltimore. If you begin to notice a pattern pointing to a potential culprit, he says, eliminate that particular food from your diet and see if your symptoms disappear as well.

Be wary of dairy. Many people develop twitchy bowels because they can't digest lactose, the sugar in milk, explains Melvyn Werbach, M.D., a physician in Los Angeles who specializes in nutritional medicine and the author of *Healing with Food*. You might try giving up milk and milk products for a while to see if your symptoms clear up, he suggests.

If you just can't bear the thought of sitting down to a bowl of dry cereal in the morning, consider taking a lactase supplement (such as Lactaid) instead, Dr. Werbach says. This product, which is sold in grocery and drugstores, contains an enzyme that helps your gut break down lactose. You mix it directly into your milk or you can take it right before you eat a dairy food.

Don't forgo fiber. Perhaps the last thing you would think of feeding an angry bowel is fiber. Yet a high-fiber diet can actually help relieve the intestinal spasms of IBS by slightly distending the colon. It may also relieve constipation, another common IBS symptom, by retaining water in the stool.

To increase your fiber intake, Dr. Werbach suggests gradually adding more whole-grain breads and cereals and more fresh fruits and vegetables to your diet. You can also take a fiber supplement that contains psyllium (such as Metamucil) or methylcellulose (such as Citrucel).

Be aware that eating more fiber can temporarily aggravate IBS by producing more gas. This usually subsides in just a few weeks.

Capitalize on carbs. Fill your diet with complex carbohydrates such as pasta, rice, fruits, and vegetables, while trimming the fat as much as possible. Fatty foods, especially meats, can send your intestines into spasms.

Think small. Feasting on a five-course spread can tax your intestines and lead to cramping and diarrhea. So eat smaller but more frequent meals—say, six mini-meals spread throughout the day rather than the standard three squares—or switch to smaller portions.

Avoid caffeine and nicotine. Because cigarettes and caffeinated drinks such as coffee, tea, and cola act as stimulants, they may irritate your bowel and aggravate IBS symptoms, says Dr. Schuster.

Mind your dining. "Take your meals without distractions, worries, and interruptions," suggests Brian Rees, M.D., medical director of the Maharishi Ayur-Veda Medical Center in Pacific Palisades, California. The idea is to focus on your eating, he says. "If your attention is drawn to something besides your food, you can develop indigestion, gas, bloating, and cramping."

Learn to relax. Since stress can make IBS symptoms even worse, learning to take it easy may ease your discomfort. In particular, "if you're a Type A personality, aim for an A-minus instead," Dr. Schuster says. Relaxation tapes can help, as can books on coping and stress-management techniques.

Kidney Stones

S ome wags have suggested that kidney stones are nature's way of allowing men to experience what it feels like to give birth. Indeed, the pain is said to be just as intense—and there is great rejoicing when the little devil finally makes its way to the outside world.

A kidney stone is actually a crystallized mass of minerals that forms, as you might expect, in the kidneys. Stones can range from mi croscopic to almond size. The small ones pass through the bladder and out in the urine without incident. The larger ones can lodge in the ureters, the narrow passageways that carry urine from the kidneys to the bladder. When that happens, every cell in your body will resonate with the message "Get me to an emergency room!"

About 10 percent of people develop kidney stones at some point in their lifetimes. Most of these unfortunate folks—about four of every five, by one estimate—are men. And once you pass one stone, there is a 50-50 chance that you'll form another one within five to seven years.

Skipping Stones

A kidney stone often produces such intolerable pain that it will drive you to seek medical attention without delay. And that's exactly what you should do, experts say. Your stone needs to be analyzed—and you need to undergo some tests, too. The results will help your doctor determine what kind of chemical imbalance caused your stone. Preventive measures can then be prescribed to stop more stones from forming.

Only time—and a whole lot of fluids—will bring your stone to pass. But the following strategies will help ensure that this painful pebble is your first and last.

When to See the Doctor

A kidney stone typically produces pain that is so sudden and so intense that you will most likely head for the nearest emergency room. "You'll almost always feel it in your side, between your ribs and your hip," says Dudley Danoff, M.D., senior attending urologist at Cedars–Sinai Medical Center in Los Angeles. The pain can radiate into the groin area as well.

With some kidney stones, though, the pain isn't as severe as it is persistent. And if the stone is situated low in the urinary tract, you may feel a need to urinate constantly. Either of these symptoms should be checked out by your doctor.

You should also see your doctor if you notice blood in your urine, advises John Birkhoff, M.D., assistant professor of clinical urology at Columbia–Presbyterian Medical Center in New York City. "It could be a stone, but it could also be an infection or a tumor," he explains.

Eat less meat. A diet high in animal protein predisposes you to the formation of calcium stones, says John Birkhoff, M.D., assistant professor of clinical urology at Columbia–Presbyterian Medical Center in New York City. So if you're prone to stones, it is a good idea to reduce your meat intake.

Shake the salt habit. A diet that is high in sodium can also set you up for stones. "Don't add salt to your food," advises Dr. Birkhoff. "And you should avoid eating highly salted foods such as potato chips."

Ferret out fat. "When dietary fat isn't fully absorbed from the gut, it can contribute to the formation of kidney stones by binding with calcium," says Melvyn Werbach, M.D., a physician in Los Angeles who specializes in nutritional medicine and the author of *Healing with Food.* Now you have yet another good reason to keep your fat intake in check.

Be fluent in fluids. "Never pass a water fountain without taking a drink," urges Dudley Danoff, M.D., senior attending urologist at Cedars–Sinai Medical Center in Los Angeles. "A big stone starts from a little pebble. If you're well-hydrated, you'll pass the little pebble before it evolves into a big stone."

How much fluid do you need? Aim for at least eight 8-ounce glasses of water a day. If you feel as though you are becoming water-logged, just remember that a high fluid intake can reduce your odds of a subsequent stone by 30 percent.

Exercise caution. "If you work out, you can dehydrate very quickly," says Fred L. Coe, M.D., chief of the nephrology section at the University of Chicago School of Medicine. "Be extra careful to drink a lot of fluids when you exercise, especially in hot weather."

Beware the "stone belt." There are certain regions of the country where kidney stones tend to be quite common. "It's related to the mineral content of the local water supply and the amount of humidity in the air," explains Dr. Danoff. He suggests contacting a nearby hospital and asking if you're in a so-called stone belt. "If the local water contains high amounts of calcium or certain mineral salts, you might be better off drinking bottled water," he adds.

Eschew the booze. People who are prone to stones consume almost twice as much alcohol as people who aren't, according to Dr. Werbach. If you drink, do so in moderation.

Decide on decaf. "We don't yet know whether caffeine increases the risk of developing kidney stones," Dr. Werbach says. "But we do know that it substantially increases the amount of calcium in the urine." And all that extra calcium becomes available for stone formation.

Keep an eye on oxalate. "If tests show that the amount of oxalate in your urine is high, you may be able to cut your risk of kidney stones by limiting your intake of high-oxalate foods," says Dr. Werbach. Among the foods you'll want to avoid are beans, cocoa, instant coffee, tea, parsley, rhubarb, and spinach.

Take care with calcium. If your body doesn't metabolize calcium properly to begin with, you could make yourself more susceptible to developing kidney stones by eating a high-calcium diet. "There are benefits to calcium, so you don't want to limit your intake excessively unless there is too much of the mineral in your urine," Dr. Birkhoff says.

He recommends consuming one portion of milk product each day—a glass of milk, a small wedge of hard cheese, a scoop of soft cheese, or a moderate amount of yogurt. "Add that to the calcium you get from other foods, and you should be averaging 800 to 900 milligrams a day," Dr. Birkhoff says. "That's a reasonable amount. What you don't want is excess."

Knee Pain

Imagine, for a moment, life without knees. You couldn't drive a car or ride a bicycle or climb a flight of stairs. And how would your doctor test your reflexes—by hitting you on the elbow with his little mallet?

Without question, knees do have certain advantages. But they are also prone to problems. Once you get beneath the kneecap, the joint is really nothing more than a mass of tendons and ligaments holding together the thighbone and shinbone, with cartilage sandwiched in between. This design is much too fragile and unstable for the punishment that knees must routinely endure.

Sports such as running, skiing, and basketball do their share of damage to delicate knees. But even everyday activities such as scrubbing floors can cause problems. (This condition even has a name: housemaid's knee.)

When knees hurt, it's most often a sign of overuse syndrome, says Paul Lotke, M.D., professor of orthopedic surgery at the University of Pennsylvania Medical Center in Philadelphia. "It happens when an active person thinks he's as conditioned as he was in high school or college and does things he's not in shape for." The result is a sore knee that aches most when you bend it or when you stand up after sitting for a long time.

Knees also suffer fractures, sprains, and bruises. The cartilage that cushions them tears, and the tendons that support them become inflamed. In addition, they are a common target of arthritis.

Battling a Wounded Knee

If you injure your knee in a fall or an accident, experts recommend that you have it examined by your doctor to make sure no serious structural damage has occurred. But for knee pain that's caused by general overuse, proper self-care should do the trick. The following tips can help.

Give it a big chill. Knee pain will diminish with applications of ice, says Thomas Rizzo, Jr., M.D., a physiatrist in the department of physical medicine and rehabilitation at the Mayo Clinic in Jacksonville, Florida. "Put an ice pack on your knee for 20 minutes every couple of hours—no more frequently than that," he says. Be sure to lay the pack on a towel, not directly on your skin.

For chronic pain, rub an ice cube around your knee after any activity that makes the joint sore, suggests William S. Case, president of Case Physical Therapy in Houston.

Medicate the pain. Dr. Lotke recommends taking an over-the-counter pain reliever to soothe a sore knee. Aspirin, ibuprofen, acetaminophen, and naproxen (Aleve) can all help, he says. Choose the one that works best for you. Always read the label to determine the correct dosage.

Think twice about a brace. "Sometimes a knee brace can help, but it depends on what the problem is," Dr. Rizzo says. "Don't use one without consulting your doctor first." A brace won't cure whatever is causing your pain. But it can increase your awareness of your knee so that you're more careful not to aggravate it, according to Dr. Rizzo.

Add support to your shoe. An over-the-counter shoe insert can help relieve pain by taking pressure off your knee, Dr. Rizzo says. "It's especially helpful if you have fallen arches or you overpronate," he notes. (Overpronation means you tend to walk and stand on the inside of your foot more than you are supposed to.)

Cut back. "Limit any activity that might aggravate your knee," Dr. Lotke advises. Obviously, you'll want to restrict your participation in running and other bone-jarring sports—at least temporarily. But you should also avoid prolonged sitting, and opt for elevators and escalators over stairs.

When to See the Doctor

Any knee pain that is intermittent or clearly associated with overuse can usually be managed with self-care, says Thomas Rizzo, Jr., M.D., a physiatrist in the department of physical medicine and rehabilitation at the Mayo Clinic in Jacksonville, Florida. But, experts say, there are a number of circumstances that should alert you to visit your doctor, including the following symptoms.

- Severe swelling
- Pain when you're at rest
- Pain that radiates from your knee up to your back or down to your foot
- Difficulty straightening your knee
- Difficulty bearing weight on your knee

A fall or an accident that causes persistent, severe localized pain should also send you to your doctor, says Paul Lotke, M.D., professor of orthopedic surgery at the University of Pennsylvania Medical Center in Philadelphia. You could have structural damage in the joint itself, such as a cartilage or ligament tear.

Sit pretty. When it comes to knee pain, it's not only how long you sit but also the way you sit that can cause problems, says Ed Laskowski, M.D., co-director of the Sportsmedicine Center at the Mayo Clinic in Rochester, Minnesota. In particular, be wary of any position in which your knees are very flexed. "If you have to sit for a long time, find a way to straighten your leg to disengage the kneecap from its groove and relieve the pressure," he advises.

Don't lock up. Locking your knees puts unwelcome pressure on an already-aching joint, Dr. Lotke says. "Try bending your knees just a little when you stand," he suggests. "At first you'll feel as though you're squatting, even if you've moved only a fraction of an inch. But if you look at yourself in a mirror, you won't even notice it. The more you do it, the easier it will become—it's much better for your knees in the long run."

Lose the limp. If you can't walk without limping, you should use crutches or a cane, Dr. Rizzo says. Otherwise, you're increasing the workload for muscles and tendons elsewhere in your body, and that can cause problems.

Take baby steps. Once your knee is feeling better, return to your normal routine gradually, advises Phillip A. Bauman, M.D., clinical instructor in orthopedic surgery at the Columbia University College of Physicians and Surgeons and associate attending physician of orthopedic surgery at St. Luke's/Roosevelt Hospital Center, both in New York City. "You should experience no pain at all when going about your daily tasks before you try to do something more stressful, like play a sport," he says.

When you feel as though you're ready to take on a more strenuous activity, discontinue any painkillers that you may have been taking. That way, you'll know if you're overdoing it because the medication isn't masking your pain, Dr. Bauman explains.

Upsize your thighs. You can protect your knee against future injury by strengthening the thigh muscles known as the quadriceps, experts say. These two exercises can help.

- Dr. Laskowski suggests lunges: Step forward, bending the lead leg at the knee. Keep the back leg straighter. Hold for about 10 seconds. Return to the starting position, then repeat with the other leg. Do three sets of 12 to 15 repetitions per leg every other day, he says.
- Case recommends one-quarter squats: Stand about 1½ feet from a wall, then lean back against it. Slowly slide down the wall, bending your knees as you lower yourself 4 to 6 inches. Hold this position for 5 to 10 seconds, then push yourself back up the wall. "You should feel a stretch just above your kneecaps," Case says. "If you feel pain below your kneecaps, you've gone too far." Start with 10 repetitions and build up to 35 repetitions, twice a day.

Become a pedal pusher. To stay in shape while protecting your knee, nothing beats a session on a stationary bicycle, experts say. "Your knee can tolerate the range of motion that pedaling puts it through, and there's no impact," Dr. Laskowski notes. "It also gives a good workout to the inner portion of the quadriceps."

Be sure to set the bicycle's tension at medium so that it causes no discomfort in your knees, Case says. He also recommends adjusting the seat so that your knees are slightly bent when the pedals are closest to the ground.

Menstrual Pain

S ome people blame it all on Eve. If she had shown just a little more restraint in the Garden of Eden, they say, you might not have to suffer through the monthly ritual of cramps, headaches, and bloating—not to mention nausea and diarrhea—that your mother (and probably your grandmother) affectionately referred to as the curse.

The assorted aches and pains that accompany the arrival of your period every 28 days or so are the result of a series of hormonal changes that prepare your body for pregnancy. When you don't conceive, your body discharges the unfertilized egg as well as the blood-laden uterine lining (called the endometrium). Incidentally, it only seems as though you're bleeding gallons: The actual amount of blood lost every month averages about 2 ounces.

While the menstrual cycle may be a fact of life, menstrual pain is not. "It's not necessarily 'normal,' even though your mother may have told you it is," says David Olive, M.D., chief of reproductive endocrinology and infertility at Yale University School of Medicine. "And you don't have to just live with it."

Still, that is exactly what many women do. Perhaps it is because menstrual pain diminishes with time: Cramps, for example, appear to be much more common among younger women than among older women. And of course, once you reach menopause, they disappear completely.

No More Pain, Period

Menstrual pain tends to subside after the first day or two of your period. But that doesn't mean that you have to feel miserable for those 48 hours. Try these tips for fast relief.

Work up a sweat. Okay, so you probably don't feel like exercising just now. But give it a try, because it can do you a world of good. The reason is that exercise steps up the production of endorphins, which are your body's natural painkillers, according to Norman Schulman, M.D., an obstetrician/gynecologist at Cedars–Sinai Medical Center in Los Angeles.

"If moving around hurts, try lifting weights or riding a stationary bicycle—any activity that won't jostle you around too much," advises Lisa Rarick, M.D., director of the division of reproductive and urological drug products at the Food and Drug Administration. "And try to exercise regularly before your period. It may help reduce your discomfort."

Try to relax. Practicing a relaxation technique can help you manage any kind of pain, Dr. Schulman says. Choose imagery, meditation, yoga—or just take long walks. "Find something that works for you," he suggests.

Keep warm. "Don't let your body get cold," urges Felice Dunas, Ph.D., a licensed acupuncturist and a doctor of clinical Chinese medicine in private practice in Topanga, California. "According to the principles of Chinese medicine, cold causes muscle contractions and spasms. Heat, on the other hand, can lessen the severity of cramping."

"Moist heat is best—a hot bath, a hot-water bottle, or a heating pad that circulates warm water," adds Dr. Olive. Whichever treatment method you choose, use it as often as necessary, he says.

Stay away from sweets. Sugary foods can increase your body's production of prostaglandins, according to Cynthia M. Watson, M.D., a family practitioner in private practice in Santa Monica, California. Prostaglandins are hormonelike fatty acids that can contribute to cramping.

Opt for homeopathy. The homeopathic remedy Magnesia phosphorica can help relieve menstrual cramps, Dr. Watson says. She recommends taking four 6C tablets three or four times a day, beginning a couple of days before your period and continuing until your cramps subside. (The notation 6C refers to the remedy's potency,

When to See the Doctor

Menstrual pain usually subsides on its own with time. But certain changes should be brought to your doctor's attention, advises Norman Schulman, M.D., an obstetrician/gynecologist at Cedars–Sinai Medical Center in Los Angeles. These include the following symptoms.

- Heavier or irregular bleeding
- Localized pain that does not go away when your period is over
- Disabling pain
- Pain accompanied by fever

You should also see your doctor if you have severe pelvic discomfort at times other than your period—especially if it's accompanied by an aching lower back, painful bowel movements, or painful intercourse. These symptoms could signal the onset of endometriosis, an overgrowth of the uterine lining that sometimes results in infertility.

which is indicated on the label.) You'll find Magnesia phosphorica in health food stores and wherever homeopathic remedies are sold.

Sample a supplement. Supplements of the amino acid DL phenylalanine can help ease menstrual cramps, according to Hyla Cass, M.D., assistant clinical professor of psychiatry at the University of California, Los Angeles, UCLA School of Medicine. You might find the amino acid in capsule form in health food stores, or you can ask your pharmacist if he can get it for you. "Follow the directions on the bottle for proper dosage," she advises.

Help yourself to herbs. The herbs yarrow and fenugreek can help maintain hormonal balance during your period, according to Pamela Miller, a licensed acupuncturist at Balfour Chiropractic in Northridge, California. Both are natural sources of progesterone, the hormone that causes the uterine lining to thicken. Miller suggests steeping either herb in boiling water and then drinking the tea once a day for the duration of your period. Yarrow and fenugreek are available in most health food stores.

Say yes to progesterone. Experts recommend applying a 3 percent natural progesterone cream to your thighs, abdomen, and breasts (the areas of your body with the most fatty tissue) starting on day 14 of your cycle and continuing until the day your period starts.

Note: This is not the same as the yam-derived creams usually sold in health food stores. If you can't find natural progesterone cream in your area, you can order it by mail from Transitions for Health, 621 S.W. Alder Street, Suite 900, Portland, OR 97205-3627

Get aid from NSAIDs. Nonsteroidal anti-inflammatory drugs (NSAIDs) neutralize pain-producing prostaglandins, according to Emanuel Fliegelman, D.O., professor emeritus of obstetrics and gynecology at the Philadelphia College of Osteopathic Medicine. He recommends ibuprofen or naproxen (Aleve).

If you opt for one of these over-the-counter medications, you can maximize its therapeutic benefits by taking it at the right time. "NSAIDs are most helpful when you start taking them one to two days before your period, and then continue through your period," says Lisa Barrie Schwartz, M.D., assistant professor of obstetrics and gynecology at New York University Medical Center in New York City.

Migraine

There is headache, and there is migraine. One is a fingernail screeching down a blackboard, the other, a dozen jackhammers chewing up the street outside your window. One is the crackle of a firecracker, the other, the blast of a stick of dynamite. One is . . . well, you get the idea.

The word *migraine* is derived from the Greek *hemicrania,* which, loosely translated, means half a head. It alludes to the fact that a migraine typically affects only one side of the face, usually around the eye. The pain is often described as throbbing or pulsating and may be accompanied by nausea, vomiting, and extreme sensitivity to light and sound.

Sometimes a migraine is preceded by an aura—visual distortions such as blurred vision and zigzagging lights. This "announcement" of a migraine's pending arrival is never welcome: It foretells incapacitating pain that can last anywhere from a few hours to several days.

Scientists can't yet explain why or how a migraine occurs. They do know that it can be triggered by foods, stress, pollutants, changes in the weather, and disrupted eating and sleeping patterns. Hormones appear to play a role, too: Women are twice as likely as men to suffer from chronic migraines, and most of them get hit during their menstrual periods.

Make Gains on Migraine Pain

To manage migraines effectively, you must take steps to prevent attacks and to minimize pain when one does occur. Here is what the experts advise.

When to See the Doctor

Consult your doctor if you have recurrent headaches of any kind, experts say. If you are diagnosed as having migraines, then be alert for these symptoms, which require immediate medical attention.

- Attacks that become more frequent or severe
- Pain that lasts for more than 12 hours
- Vision changes
- Tingling, numbness, or weakness in one arm

Lie low. Migraine pain is very easily aggravated by physical activity—even something as mild as walking or bending over. "When migraines strike, most people want to crawl into a dark corner and be left alone," says Robert Kunkel, M.D., staff physician at the Headache Center of the Cleveland Clinic Foundation. The truth is, that may not be a bad idea.

Get some shut-eye. Sleep almost always helps relieve migraine pain, experts agree. But rather than lying down, position yourself so that your upper body is elevated at about a 45-degree angle, suggests R. Michael Gallagher, D.O., director of the University Headache Center at the University of Medicine and Dentistry of New Jersey School of Osteopathic Medicine in Stratford. "You want your head to be higher than your heart," he explains. Sitting in a recliner will work well.

Go for cold. It has long been theorized that a migraine occurs when blood vessels in the brain rapidly constrict and then dilate. "A cold pack can make the blood vessels constrict again," says Dr. Gallagher. He suggests that you try wrapping some ice or a ready-made pack—the kind that wraps around your neck and the back of your head—in a towel and applying it to your neck and head. "During an attack, you can leave the pack on for an extended period of time," he says.

Touch your temples. "If you have throbbing pain in your temples, applying pressure can help relieve it," according to Dr. Kunkel. He suggests either wrapping a bandanna around your head and tying it tight or massaging the area with your fingertips. Just be extremely careful: Your temples are probably very tender.

Keep tabs on your triggers. Maintaining a food diary can help you identify the foods that set off your migraine attacks, Dr. Kunkel says. He suggests writing down everything you eat as well as when your migraines occur. "After two or three attacks, you'll probably notice a pattern," he explains. "A migraine usually sets in within 6 to 24 hours after eating a particular food."

Here are common triggers that you should watch out for.
- Tyramine, found in cheese, chicken livers, sour cream, and red wine
- Phenylethylamine, found mainly in chocolate
- Nitrates, which are added to meats as preservatives
- Lactose, found in milk and milk products (particularly likely to trigger migraines if you are lactose intolerant.)
- Caffeine, found in coffee, tea, and some soft drinks
- Aspartame, an artificial sweetener (brand name NutraSweet) that is used in some low-calorie foods

Pass on MSG. The flavor enhancer monosodium glutamate (MSG) is also a common food trigger. But it deserves special mention because people tend to associate it solely with Chinese takeout. In fact, it's found in a variety of canned, frozen, and prepared foods, sometimes listed as protein hydrolyzate or calcium caseinate. "A large number of migraine patients are susceptible to MSG," says Seymour Diamond, M.D., director of the Diamond Headache Clinic in Chicago and author of *The Hormone Headache*. "They develop headaches within 15 to 30 minutes after eating a food flavored with just a small amount of MSG."

Eat on time. "Maintaining a regular diet is very important," Dr. Gallagher says. "Migraines are associated with blood vessel changes, and these changes happen much more readily when your blood sugar level shifts."

A Prescription for Your Pain

If self-care options are no match for your migraines, your doctor may recommend managing your condition with medicine. He will prescribe either prophylactic (preventive) or abortive medication, depending on the frequency and severity of your attacks. "Prophylactic drugs are taken on a daily basis, while abortive drugs are taken only when a migraine occurs," explains Jerome Goldstein, M.D., assistant clinical professor of neurology at the University of California, San Francisco, School of Medicine and director of the San Francisco Headache Clinic.

The most highly regarded abortive medicine is sumatriptan (Imitrex), which works rapidly to short-circuit migraine symptoms. Originally available only by injection, it now comes in pill form as well. Prophylactic drugs include beta-blockers, calcium channel blockers, and nonsteroidal anti-inflammatory drugs (NSAIDs).

Your doctor may also prescribe a strong narcotic to take only when all other medications fail. In addition, you may be given an anti-emetic to combat nausea and vomiting, which are frequent sidekicks to migraine pain.

Eschew alcohol. If you are prone to migraines, don't drink, Dr. Diamond urges. "Alcohol—especially red wine (which contains tyramine)—can provoke an attack," he says.

Evaluate your estrogen intake. In women, migraines have been linked to monthly hormonal fluctuations. If you're prone to attacks and you're taking birth control pills or hormone replacement therapy—both of which contain estrogen—Dr. Diamond suggests talking to your doctor about adjusting your dosage. "Usually estrogen increases the frequency, duration, severity, and complications of migraines," he notes.

Stay calm. Uncontrolled stress and anxiety can also invite a migraine attack, experts say. "Make sure that you allow some time every day to do whatever relaxes you, even if it's only for ½ hour in the evening," Dr. Gallagher urges. "Don't just go to work and go to bed."

Bank on biofeedback. "Biofeedback is a form of conditioning in which you learn how to automatically warm your hands and relax the muscles around your head and neck," explains Jerome Goldstein, M.D., assistant clinical professor of neurology at the University of California, San Francisco, School of Medicine and director of the San Francisco Headache Clinic. "This helps reduce the frequency and severity of migraine attacks."

Biofeedback machines, which monitor various vital signs, are available for home use. But experts advise consulting a professional for training in the proper use of these devices.

Stick to a schedule. Get up at the same time every day of the week, including Saturdays and Sundays. When you sleep in, you're messing with your body's internal clock, Dr. Gallagher explains. Your body revs up certain metabolic processes later than it should, and that can set the stage for a migraine—just in time to ruin your weekend.

Mind your magnesium level. "People are more prone to migraine attacks when they're marginally deficient in magnesium," according to Melvyn Werbach, M.D., a physician in Los Angeles who specializes in nutritional medicine and the author of *Healing with Food.* He recommends taking 200 milligrams of the mineral every day for two months to see if it has any impact on the number of migraines you experience.

Note: People who have heart or kidney problems should not take supplemental magnesium.

Fish around for relief. "Studies have shown that people suffering from severe, chronic migraines have fewer attacks and less pain once they start using fish oil supplements," Dr. Werbach says. He recommends cholesterol-free fish oil extract, which is rich in omega-3 fatty acids. Take 3 grams of the extract (available in drugstores and health food stores) three times a day for a trial period of three to six weeks, he says—but only in consultation with your doctor.

Consider aspirin. A large-scale study of 20,000 physicians that found aspirin to be effective in preventing heart disease also suggested that the drug may have similar effects on migraines. "A number of the study participants were migraine sufferers," Dr. Diamond notes. "Those who took one baby aspirin a day experienced a significant reduction in the number and severity of migraine attacks." Could an aspirin a day keep your migraines at bay? He suggests discussing it with your physician.

Prevent period pain. If you're a woman whose migraines follow your menstrual cycle, Dr. Kunkel recommends taking an anti-inflammatory such as ibuprofen starting two to three days before your period and continuing through your period. "It can reduce the severity of a migraine or even stop it from coming," he says.

Prepare for travel. A migraine is sometimes associated with a change in altitude, Dr. Kunkel says. So if you are planning to fly somewhere—or do anything at high elevations, such as skiing—he suggests taking Diamox (a prescription diuretic with the active ingredient acetazolamide) a couple of days beforehand. "We're not sure exactly why, but it often reduces the severity of a headache," he says. "Diamox is a little different chemically from other diuretics."

Muscle Cramps

T alk about a rude awakening. Your peaceful slumber is suddenly disrupted by the feeling that someone has your calf in a vise and won't stop tightening the grip. Yikes—a cramp! Yanked from dreamland by the agonizing pain, you perch on the edge of your bed and massage the muscle for what seems like an eternity. At last the pain subsides. But when will it strike again?

Cramps do seem to have a special affinity for the calves—but other parts of your body are just as vulnerable. Your neck, back, thighs, and feet can also fall victim to these abnormal, agonizing muscle contractions.

A whole host of factors have been linked to the onset of cramps. One common culprit is muscle fatigue, says John Cianca, M.D., assistant professor of physical medicine and rehabilitation at Baylor College of Medicine in Houston.

Muscle fatigue tends to occur when you overexert yourself— for example, by walking or running harder or farther than you normally do. "Your muscles aren't getting enough nutrients, so they run out of gas," Dr. Cianca explains. "Waste products build up, and the electrolyte balance—which controls the contraction of muscles—is offset."

All of this sets the stage for the tightening, clenching, squeezing sensations that are a cramp's trademarks. They may come on during physical activity—or they may be delayed until long afterward. "You might move funny while you're lying in bed, and the muscle contracts. It's because the muscle is already fatigued," Dr. Cianca says.

Cramps may also crop up when a muscle is overstretched or strained or takes a direct blow. Other potential triggers include mineral depletion, impaired circulation, and sudden changes in temperature.

When to See the Doctor

In most cases, a cramp is a minor, isolated event. But you should seek medical attention if you notice any of the following symptoms, says Myles J. Schneider, D.P.M., a podiatrist in Annandale, Virginia, and co-author of *The Athlete's Health Care Book.*
- Cramping continues to occur, becoming more frequent or intense.
- You experience persistent swelling or discoloration.
- The area of the cramp feels warm to the touch compared with the same area of the unaffected leg (or whatever muscle group is involved).
- The cramp is accompanied by a low-grade fever.
- You have extreme pain when you move the affected area.

Uncramp Your Style

On rare occasions a cramp can become so intense that it actually tears some muscle fibers. For the most part, though, it's not a serious health problem.

But that doesn't mean that you should leave it alone—even if the pain would allow you to. "The longer a muscle stays in a tight, spasmodic condition, the greater the potential for injury," Dr. Cianca says.

The next time a cramp catches you off guard, here's what you can do to relieve the pain.

Call it quits. If you get a cramp while moving around, "stop what you're doing—or at least slow down," says Dr. Cianca. "If you're running, for example, slow to a walk."

Counter the contraction. You can gently relax a cramped muscle by guiding it through its normal range of motion, says Myles J. Schneider, D.P.M., a podiatrist in Annandale, Virginia, and co-author of *The Athlete's Health Care Book.* For a cramp in your calf, he suggests

Stretch It Out

A few minutes of stretching before a workout or any strenuous activity just may be your best insurance policy against cramps. These gentle exercises help limber up your muscles and prime them for the hard work that lies ahead.

- For your calves, William S. Case, president of Case Physical Therapy in Houston, suggests this stretch: Stand facing a wall. Place your palms on the wall and lean toward it, with one leg forward and one leg back. Your forward leg should be bent at the knee. You should feel a pulling sensation in the calf of the back leg as you lower your heel toward the ground. Hold for 10 to 20 seconds and repeat five times.
- For your thighs, try this stretch recommended by John Cianca, M.D., assistant professor of physical medicine and rehabilitation at Baylor College of Medicine in Houston: Lie on your back with both legs outstretched. Lift one leg straight up, flexing from your hip. Pull that leg toward your head, holding it wherever you feel the stretch. If you can't reach your leg, he suggests looping a towel over your foot and grabbing the ends with your hands. Hold the stretch for 30 to 60 seconds. "You should feel tension, but it shouldn't hurt," Dr. Cianca says.
- For your feet, Myles J. Schneider, D.P.M., a podiatrist in Annandale, Virginia, and co-author of *The Athlete's Health Care Book,* recommends this stretch: Sit or lie down with your legs outstretched so that your weight is off your feet. Point your toes as far as you can, then flex them toward your head as far as you can. Hold for 10 seconds, when your toes are pointed toward your nose, and repeat 5 to 10 times.

holding your calf with one hand while pulling your foot toward you with the other hand. The same instructions apply for a cramp in your foot—just place your hand in the arch of your foot instead of on your calf. In both cases hold the stretch until you feel the cramp release.

Rub yourself the right way. Massage the calf, arch, and toes with baby oil for 5 minutes, using a back-and-forth motion, across the length of the muscle, Dr. Schneider suggests. Rolling over the affected muscle from side to side with the palms of your hands can also help, he says.

Cool it. Applying ice to a muscle can relieve any cramp-related soreness and swelling, Dr. Cianca says. He recommends freezing water in a plastic-foam cup, then tearing a strip from the cup to expose the ice and rubbing the ice directly on the affected area. Start gently, and as the area gets colder, press a little harder. Continue for 10 to 15 minutes.

Take a painkiller. If you're still very sore after the cramp has subsided, an over-the-counter pain reliever might be in order. "Take two aspirin immediately and two more after 4 hours," advises Dr. Schneider.

Turn up the heat. For recurring cramps, Dr. Schneider recommends regular applications of moist heat to the affected muscle. Warm the muscle for 10 to 15 minutes, five or six times a day. "Continue the applications every day until there is no trace of cramping," he says.

Fill up with fluids. Keeping yourself adequately hydrated can help prevent cramps. Be sure to top off your tank before and during any physical activity—especially if you're working up a sweat in hot weather. "You should drink 8 to 12 ounces of fluid before you start exercising," says Brent S. E. Rich, M.D., staff physician at Arizona Orthopaedic and Sports Medicine Specialists in Phoenix and team physician at Arizona State University in Tempe. "Follow up with 4 to 8 ounces of fluid every 30 to 45 minutes while you're working out."

Be a sport. "If you're low in sodium or potassium, you might be prone to cramping," Dr. Rich says. The reason is that both minerals are electrolytes, which regulate muscle contractions (among other important bodily functions). Sports drinks such as Gatorade, he notes, can help replenish your supply of sodium and potassium. He recommends diluting the drink with a little water, so that your body absorbs it better.

Prize potassium. To help maintain your body's levels of muscle-friendly potassium, be sure to eat lots of foods rich in the mineral, advises Melvyn Werbach, M.D., a physician in Los Angeles who specializes in nutritional medicine and the author of *Healing with Foods.* Bananas are the top choice. Other good sources include apricots, potatoes, cantaloupe, and spinach.

Up your C level. Increasing your intake of vitamin C can help keep your muscles from cramping, says Dr. Schneider. His recommendation: timed-release vitamin C capsules taken twice a day—1,000 milligrams in the morning, 1,000 milligrams at night.

Note: Some people may experience diarrhea when taking more than 1,200 milligrams of vitamin C a day.

Toe the line on pain. If your calf muscles are susceptible to recurring cramps, they're probably weak, says Dr. Cianca. You can build them up with simple strengthening exercises. He recommends toe raises: Simply rise up on your toes, hold for 5 seconds, then return your heels to the floor. Repeat 15 to 20 times, two or three times a day. To enhance the benefits of this exercise, you may want to try holding dumbbells at your shoulders, he says.

Hang loose. When you're exercising, make sure that nothing is too tight, says Dr. Schneider. This includes clothing as well as elastic bandages and wraps.

Take it easy. Since cramps often result from overexertion, weekend warriors are highly susceptible. Dr. Cianca urges common sense. "Don't overdo it," he says. "It's a matter of being physically prepared for what you're going to do."

Muscle Spasms

Y ou might think of a muscle spasm as a cramp that overstays its welcome. While a cramp usually relaxes its grip in a matter of minutes once you rest the affected muscle, a spasm can produce days of unrelenting pain and soreness.

"A spasm doesn't just go away when you straighten the muscle," says William S. Case, president of Case Physical Therapy in Houston. And it can strike just about anywhere in the body: The neck, the back, the legs, and even the fingers are vulnerable.

"In lay terms, *spasm* means that a muscle or muscle group gets very tight," explains John Cianca, M.D., assistant professor of physical medicine and rehabilitation at Baylor College of Medicine in Houston. "It hurts when you try to move into certain positions." A spasm in your back, for example, can make bending forward an excruciating endeavor.

For some people, a spasm may signal the existence of an underlying health problem, such as an injury or a neurological disorder. More likely, though, it's the result of overexertion—"like when a weekend athlete with weak muscles overdoes it," says Case.

Put the Squeeze on Pain

It takes time for a spasm to subside. But there is a lot you can do to ease your discomfort and speed the healing process. Here's what experts recommend.

Baby your body. The affected muscles need rest. You can ease their workload by positioning your body in a way that allows them to relax, Dr. Cianca says. "If you have a back spasm, for example, the best thing that you can do is lie down. Standing requires the muscles to work harder."

When to See the Doctor

Any significant bleeding or bruising in the area of a spasm requires prompt medical attention, says Brent S. E. Rich, M.D., staff physician at Arizona Orthopaedic and Sports Medicine Specialists in Phoenix and team physician at Arizona State University in Tempe. You should also see your doctor if the spasm is in your leg and you're having trouble walking.

If you develop a recurrent spasm or if a spasm lasts for more than a few days, your doctor or a physical therapist may be able to work the muscle to relax it and restore its normal function, says John Cianca, M.D., assistant professor of physical medicine and rehabilitation at Baylor College of Medicine in Houston.

Get back on your feet. "You don't want to lie around and do nothing for too long," says Dr. Cianca. "Prolonged bed rest can promote muscle weakness. If your pain is so bad that you feel you have to stay in bed all the time, you should see your doctor."

Chill out. In the acute stage of a spasm, when the pain is most intense, experts advise applying ice to the affected area. Use a plastic bag filled with crushed ice or a bag of frozen peas—anything that will conform to the contour of the body at the site of the spasm, Case says. Wrap the ice pack in a towel and place it on the affected area. "Leave it on for 10 to 20 minutes and repeat two or three times a day," Case suggests.

Turn up the heat. You don't want to apply heat to a spasm right when it starts since that could increase the inflammatory response, Dr. Cianca says. But after the first 48 hours, "heat applications can help the muscle relax by increasing blood flow and getting more nutrients to it," he adds.

As a general guideline, Case suggests using heat in the morning, when the muscle is stiff, and ice later in the day, when the muscle may be sore. "Place a damp towel over a heating pad to create moist heat," he says. "Leave it on for 15 to 20 minutes and repeat two or three times a day." Hot baths and showers can also be helpful, he adds.

Rub it in. You can add massage to your treatment program after the first 48 hours. "Work the area that has the spasm," Case says. "But don't overdo it. The massage should be gentle and relaxing—no pain, no digging too deep. If you're too vigorous, the muscle will spasm again because you're hurting it."

Wrap It up. Compressing the affected area with an elastic bandage can prevent the muscle from bleeding internally, says Brent S. E. Rich, M.D., staff physician at Arizona Orthopaedic and Sports Medicine Specialists in Phoenix and team physician at Arizona State University in Tempe. "Wrap the area firmly, but not so tightly that the blood supply is reduced," he suggests. "If the area feels tingly or numb, the bandage is too tight."

Take a pain reliever. To ease your discomfort and reduce inflammation, Dr. Rich recommends taking an over-the-counter anti-inflammatory drug such as ibuprofen. "But if you feel that you need to continue taking medication after a week, see your physician," he advises.

Flex your muscle. Once the spasm starts to ease up, stretching the muscle can promote healing and help prevent a recurrence. Exactly what type of stretching you should do depends on the muscle involved. "You want to move in the opposite direction of the spasm," says Dr. Cianca. "You want to flex the muscle rather than contract it." For example, a spasm in your calf pulls your foot down, so you want to gently push your foot up. A back spasm pulls you upright, so you want to slowly bend forward.

Do your exercises after applying heat or taking a hot shower, when the muscle is loose, Case suggests. "Never stretch a cold muscle," he says. "And stretch gently—to the point where it is comfortable but doesn't hurt. If it hurts, you're overdoing it." He recommends holding each stretch for 15 to 30 seconds and repeating it no more than five times. "It's better to hold the stretch longer and do fewer repetitions," Case says.

Ease into your routine. Resume activities gradually—don't overstress the muscle as soon as the spasm goes away. "Avoid any activity that reproduces the pain," Case says. "If necessary, switch to something less challenging. If you can't go for your usual run because it hurts, then walk instead. If that goes okay, you can do a little more later on."

Be prepared. "The best way to prevent a spasm from recurring is to keep the muscle strong and flexible," says Dr. Cianca. "It should be adequately prepared for what it's going to be doing." Remember to stretch before any physical activity, and do strengthening exercises to help build the muscle up. If you're an avid athlete, you might want to check with a trainer or coach to make sure that you're using the correct body mechanics for your sport.

Neck Pain

There's no question that the human body is one amazing machine. But sometimes you just have to wonder why nature couldn't come up with a better way of attaching your head to your shoulders.

Considering your neck's anatomical responsibilities—namely, balancing that bowling ball of a cranium on your body and moving it some 600 times in an hour—you'd think it would be built as solid as a tree trunk. Instead, it is more like a fragile flower stem: Inside are seven vertebrae (known collectively as the cervical spine); dozens of muscles, ligaments, and joints; and a network of nerves that reaches all your vital organs.

With such a delicate design, your neck is exceptionally vulnerable to sprains, strains, and other injuries. Probably the best-known condition is whiplash, which occurs when your neck is abruptly thrust forward or snapped backward—usually in a rear-end collision. But neck pain can also result from a ruptured disk (disks separate the vertebrae in the spine), overuse, or even poor posture.

Nearly everyone can expect to have neck pain at some point in their lives. In one study 35 percent of the participants reported having at least one bout with neck pain in the past.

Coping with a Pain in the Neck

The good news is that between 70 and 80 percent of all aching necks get better on their own within a few hours or days, according to Scott Haldeman, M.D., D.C., Ph.D., associate clinical professor of neurology at the University of California, Irvine. To nudge your pain on its way—and to keep it from paying a return visit—give these tips a try.

Be manipulative. "A gentle massage can relax neck muscles and reduce pain," says Garth Russell, M.D., clinical professor of orthopedics at the University of Missouri—Columbia School of Medicine and senior surgeon at the Columbia Spine Center, both in Columbia. "It provides great temporary relief."

Make a good impression. Practitioners of acupressure say that you can ease your discomfort by applying pressure to two points on the back of your neck. The points are located 2 inches to either side of your spine, underneath the base of your skull. Using your thumbs, press the points simultaneously for 1 minute. Keep your eyes closed as you do. To make this easier, you may want to sit and rest your elbows on a table or a desk.

Alleviate your ache with aspirin. Nonsteroidal anti-inflammatory drugs (NSAIDs) can be effective in the treatment of neck pain, according to Dr. Haldeman. "So far, none has proved to work better than aspirin," he notes. "But whichever product you choose, take the smallest dose needed to control your pain."

Make a move. "Try not to sit in the same position for too long," Dr. Russell advises. "Looking down at a desk or staring at a computer screen all day puts a great deal of stress on your neck." His recommendation is to change positions from time to time and take a stretch break at least every 30 minutes.

Stay neutral. "When you do have to stay seated, hold your neck in a neutral position," suggests Stella Shigenaka, a physical therapist at the Institute of Progressive Physical Therapy in Los Angeles. "Don't bend it forward or tilt it back." Also, adjust your chair so that your hips and knees are at 90-degree angles when you sit, she says.

Ask for a raise. Your desk can give you a pain in the neck—and not because your In box is piled high with papers. "Your desk should come to you, not the other way around," Shigenaka explains. "If it's too low, find a way either to raise it or to bring your work closer to eye level. Don't lean forward all day." If you must lean forward, do it from your hips rather than from your back or neck, she says.

When to See the Doctor

Neck pain usually subsides on its own with proper self-care. But in rare instances, it can signal the onset of a serious health problem that requires professional care. Consult your doctor if your pain does not improve within a month or if you have suffered whiplash or another neck injury, advises Scott Haldeman, M.D., D.C., Ph.D., associate clinical professor of neurology at the University of California, Irvine. You should also seek medical attention without delay if you notice any of the following symptoms.

- Lack of coordination in your legs
- Progressive numbness or weakness in your arms
- Changes in bowel or bladder function
- Persistent fever
- Pain that is considerably worse at night

Correct your computer. If you work at a computer, make sure that the screen sits directly in front of you at eye level, Shigenaka says. It shouldn't be positioned off to one side so that you have to turn your head to view it.

Straighten up and drive right. Adjust your car seat so that you can see over the steering wheel without straining, Shigenaka advises. You shouldn't have to thrust your neck forward for a clear view of the road. Also, she says, adjust your headrest so that your neck won't snap backward if you stop suddenly or are involved in an accident.

Fix bad phone habits. "Holding a telephone receiver to your ear causes you to tilt your head slightly and kink your neck," Dr. Russell says. "Shrugging your shoulder to pin the receiver to your ear is even worse." He advises against using the phone for long periods of time. "But if you must, use a speakerphone or headphones—or at least switch ears frequently," he suggests.

Brace Yourself—Or Not

Mention "whiplash" and most people think "neck brace." The question is: Do these gadgets really work? Experts say they do—if they are used the right way and for the right reasons.

"A brace may be appropriate after surgery or with an injury such as severe whiplash," according to Garth Russell, M.D., clinical professor of orthopedics at the University of Missouri—Columbia School of Medicine and senior surgeon at the Columbia Spine Center, both in Columbia. "It allows the neck to heal properly." But if you wear a brace for too long, it can actually lengthen your recovery period. "For every week that you wear a brace, it takes a month to overcome the damage you've done," he says.

Part of the problem is that they're often used improperly, says Stella Shigenaka, a physical therapist at the Institute of Progressive Physical Therapy in Los Angeles. "A brace is intended to move and stretch the neck muscles, not to keep them static," she explains. "If it fits improperly, it can do more harm than good."

"A common error is to wear a neck brace incorrectly," adds Thomas Rizzo, Jr., M.D., a physiatrist in the department of physical medicine and rehabilitation at the Mayo Clinic in Jacksonville, Florida. "The narrow part of the brace should be worn to the front, under your chin. People often wear the wide part in the front, which raises the chin too high and strains the neck muscles."

Before you decide to wear a neck brace, talk to your doctor. If your doctor thinks you need one, it should be tailored to your condition and size. And don't leave your doctor's office without clear instructions on how and when the brace should be worn.

Good night, sleep right. Snoozing in an awkward position can leave you with a doozy of a sore neck. "Sleeping on your stomach can be a real problem, especially if you have a soft mattress," notes Mary Pullig Schatz, M.D., a pathologist and yoga instructor in

Nashville and author of *Back Care Basics*. "If you must lie this way, put a large pillow under your trunk and head."

Stay away from sedatives. While you're sound asleep, your body turns continuously to make itself more comfortable, according to Dr. Haldeman. Sedatives diminish this self-adjusting ability, so your body doesn't move around as much. As a result, you may stay in an awkward position for a long period of time and wake up with an aching neck. The same thing happens when you have been drinking or you are exceptionally fatigued.

Button up your overcoat. "Cold stiffens your muscles, including those in your neck," Dr. Haldeman says. "So when you head outside in frigid weather, keep your neck warm." Just wearing a turtleneck or a scarf can make a difference.

Shrug it off. Dr. Russell recommends shoulder rolls as an easy and effective way to increase circulation and relieve tension in your neck. To do this exercise, simply make circles with your shoulders by rolling them forward, then backward. Work both shoulders simultaneously, he says. Do this exercise whenever you feel a headache coming on or your neck muscles beginning to stiffen.

Be a head turner. You can also loosen tense neck muscles with this simple exercise, Dr. Russell says: Sit up straight and bend your head forward so that your chin rests against your chest. Slowly turn your head to the left. Look up as far as you can, as though you were trying to see directly above your head. Return your chin to your chest, then turn your head to the right. Again, look up as far as you can. Repeat three times whenever you feel tension in your neck.

Penile Pain

The very thought of injuring that most precious part of the male anatomy is enough to make most men wince with pain. Fortunately, it doesn't happen all that often.

"Nature designed the penis to be tough, resilient, and durable," says Dudley Danoff, M.D., senior attending urologist at Cedars–Sinai Medical Center in Los Angeles and author of *Superpotency.* It has no bones to break, no tendons or ligaments to sprain or tear, no joints to dislocate.

Yes, injuries can occur on occasion. For example, an erect penis can collide with a woman's pelvic bone during intercourse, causing the fibrous penile tissue to rupture. (This is what is usually referred to as a fracture.) For the most part, though, penile pain signals an underlying health problem.

Among the most common causes of penile pain is Peyronie's disease, in which the fibrous tissue within the penis thickens. "You'll feel knots developing on the surface of the penis, usually on the top part," says John J. Mulcahy, M.D., Ph.D., professor of urology at the Indiana University Medical Center in Indianapolis. "You may also notice a curving, softening, or shortening of your erection." While the pain may subside on its own in time, Peyronie's disease should be treated by a physician, Dr. Mulcahy advises.

Prostatitis, an inflammation of the prostate gland, can also produce penile pain. "The pain radiates out the urethra (the tube that carries urine from the bladder), and you'll feel a burning sensation when you urinate or ejaculate," explains Stephen Jacobs, M.D., professor of urology at the University of Maryland School of Medicine in Baltimore. "But there's nothing wrong with the penis itself." More serious conditions such as prostate enlargement and prostate cancer seldom have penile pain as a symptom, he adds.

When to See the Doctor

Any time you have prolonged or intense penile pain, you should be examined by a physician," says Dudley Danoff, M.D., senior attending urologist at Cedars–Sinai Medical Center in Los Angeles and author of *Superpotency*. "This is especially important if you find it painful to urinate or if you have any type of discharge, including blood." These symptoms may indicate the presence of a kidney stone, a sexually transmitted disease, or a tumor.

A penile fracture also requires medical attention, says John J. Mulcahy, M.D., Ph.D., professor of urology at the Indiana University Medical Center in Indianapolis. How do you know when you have one? "You'll hear a pop or snap, and the erection will go down," he explains. A fracture requires surgery—but for it to be effective, it has to be done quickly.

Put Your Pain on Hold

Penile pain is usually unsettling enough that you'll want to see your doctor to find out exactly what is going on. And that's a smart move, experts agree, because you should get a proper diagnosis. Once you know the cause of your discomfort, try these tips for fast relief.

Stay warm. Some conditions respond very well to applications of heat, according to Dr. Mulcahy. He recommends draping a heating pad over the top of your penis for 20 minutes, four times a day. Be sure to use a thin towel between the heating pad and your penis. Soaking in a sitz bath or a hot tub can also be effective, he says. Ask your doctor whether heat treatments are appropriate for your condition.

Get your blood moving. To improve circulation in the groin area and speed healing, apply heat and ice simultaneously, advises Pamela Miller, a licensed acupuncturist at Balfour Chiropractic in

Northridge, California. "Place a hot pack on your lower back and a cold pack (both wrapped in towels) on your abdomen, and leave them on for 10 to 15 minutes," she says. Then reverse the packs for your next treatment: hot in front, cold in back. Repeat the applications four times a day.

Opt for an ointment. For a minor abrasion or irritation of the penis, Dr. Danoff recommends a topical ointment (such as Neosporin). But don't expect it to get better overnight, he adds. "Your penis gets erect while you sleep, causing the wound to reopen. This prolongs the healing time."

Reach for a pain reliever. An over-the-counter painkiller may provide some relief, according to Dr. Mulcahy. "Depending on your degree of discomfort, aspirin or acetaminophen may suffice," he suggests. "If neither works, then try ibuprofen."

Pinpoint the problem. The prospect of using needles to treat penile pain may leave you a bit skittish. But practitioners of acupuncture say it works. "Certain acupuncture points in the pelvic region are very effective in relieving pain in the genitals," Miller notes. To find a qualified acupuncturist in your area, contact the referral service of your local hospital.

Try something new. If intercourse aggravates your pain, experiment with different positions. "Work with your partner to find what is most comfortable for both of you," Dr. Mulcahy advises.

Just say no. With some conditions, you may need to avoid intercourse completely until you heal. "With an abrasion, for example, you don't want to do anything that tugs on the skin," Dr. Danoff says. "Just give it a rest."

The same goes for Peyronie's disease, Dr. Mulcahy adds. "Getting an erection will make your pain worse—and having intercourse will make it worse still," he notes. "If you must have sex, be very gentle. The more aggressive you are, the more it's going to hurt."

Phantom Limb Pain

It's one of the most mysterious phenomena in medicine: Virtually every person who undergoes an amputation feels sensations that seem to come from the missing limb. It's disturbing at first, but patients tend to get used to it over time. The sensations usually go away completely within a year.

Far more troublesome is phantom limb pain, which ranges in intensity from annoying to unbearable. As many as two-thirds of all amputation patients develop this condition, particularly if they were having severe pain in the limb prior to surgery.

Phantom limb pain takes many forms. People who have experienced it describe the pain as burning, cramping, stabbing, shooting, aching, or throbbing. "Sometimes it feels like the limb is still there but in an abnormal position," says Marina Russman, M.D., an anesthesiologist and pain-management specialist in private practice in Los Angeles. "For example, it feels like the missing hand is clenched in a fist, with the nails digging into the skin of the palm."

In most cases, phantom limb pain gradually subsides on its own. But sometimes it can become chronic and increasingly severe.

When the Pain Is All Too Real

Experts cannot yet explain what causes phantom limb pain. But they do know how to ease your discomfort. Here's what they advise.

Stay comfortable. "Different situations can aggravate phantom limb pain," Dr. Russman explains. "For example, your pain may get worse with exposure to cold. If that's the case, cover the limb and keep it warm." Other circumstances can cause increased discomfort as well: letting the limb hang, going to the bathroom, even yawning.

You need to figure out what bothers you so that you can avoid it, Dr. Russman says.

Keep it under wraps. Many people say that it feels better to have the limb contained, even at night. There are several ways to do this, says Karen Andrews, M.D., a consultant in the department of physical medicine and rehabilitation at the Mayo Clinic in Rochester, Minnesota. You can wear a rigid cast that is designed to be pulled over the limb, a "stump sock" that provides compression, or an elastic bandage that is wound around the limb in a figure-eight pattern. "Ask your physician or a physical therapist to make a recommendation," Dr. Andrews suggests.

Soothe with massage. "Rubbing the end of the limb can help relieve pain," Dr. Andrews says. She suggests gentle massage for 5 to 10 minutes, twice a day. "But don't be too rough in the area of the surgical incision," she cautions.

Train it. You may want to try rubbing the end of the limb with different fabrics so that it becomes accustomed to the sensations, Dr. Andrews says. Try bedsheets, towels, clothing, and other textures.

When to See the Doctor

Most cases of phantom limb pain can be managed without medical intervention. But if your pain does not improve with time, if it intensifies, or if it disrupts your daily activities or sleep, you should consult your doctor. "It's best to start treatment as soon as possible," says Marina Russman, M.D., an anesthesiologist and pain-management specialist in private practice in Los Angeles. "The earlier the treatment, the better the prognosis."

If your pain is severe, your doctor might use regional nerve blocks. "They're administered by injection, and they can produce long periods of relief," she says. If they don't work, your doctor may surgically cut or crush a nerve to interrupt stimulation.

Are You Sure It's Phantom Limb Pain?

They produce very similar symptoms. But phantom limb pain and neuroma pain are quite different—and they require different courses of treatment.

"A neuroma results from the cutting or constant irritation of a nerve," says Karen Andrews, M.D., a consultant in the department of physical medicine and rehabilitation at the Mayo Clinic in Rochester, Minnesota. "It causes tenderness and pain in the limb."

Whereas phantom limb pain usually develops shortly after surgery, neuroma pain is more likely to occur months after amputation. "If touching a specific area of the limb reproduces the pain, it's probably a neuroma," she explains. "It can be treated by burying the nerve deeper in the soft tissue."

Use your imagination. A relaxation technique called imagery can help ease your discomfort, Dr. Andrews says. To begin, lie in bed or sit comfortably and close your eyes. Visualize an activity that you enjoyed before the amputation, she suggests. For example, if you have lost part of a leg, envision yourself riding a bicycle while pedaling with both feet or sitting at the edge of a lake and dangling the missing foot in the water. If you have lost an arm, you might imagine yourself swimming or tossing a ball. "Move the sound limb as if you were doing the activity, and visualize the motion of the missing limb," she advises.

Get relief over the counter. For mild pain, over-the-counter drugs such as ibuprofen, aspirin, and acetaminophen may help, Dr. Russman says. Ask your doctor or pharmacist to recommend an appropriate product. "If the medication doesn't work, or if your pain gets worse and you require a larger dose, let your doctor know," she advises.

Consider a prescription. Certain prescription drugs normally used to treat other conditions can relieve phantom limb pain as well. "Low doses of a tricyclic antidepressant (such as Elavil) often help," Dr. Andrews notes. "The muscle relaxant Baclofen and anti-convulsant drugs (such as Tegretol) are also effective." Ask your doctor whether one of these may be right for you.

Relieve pain from within. An electronic device called an acuscope can stimulate your body's innate healing response, according to Cynthia M. Watson, M.D., a family practitioner in private practice in Santa Monica, California. "It produces a frequency current, which helps mend nerves and rebuild tissue," she explains. You'll need to check around to find a family physician or physical therapist who uses an acuscope, she adds.

Consult a professional. If you have not yet met with a physical therapist, you may want to consider doing so. A physical therapist can help rehabilitate your limb and teach you techniques for pain management, Dr. Russman says. Ask your doctor or nearby hospital for a referral.

Pizza Burn

Pizza may very well be the first food to have a medical condition named for it. The painful singe that occurs when you bite into a steamy cheese-laden slice has earned the official moniker pizza palate syndrome.

Of course, any food that's too hot can burn the roof of your mouth or your tongue. But pizza is among the most likely culprits. "The cheese on top holds in the heat," explains Richard Price, D.M.D., clinical instructor at the Henry Goldman School of Dentistry at Boston University. "Pizza can be up to 200°F when you put it in your mouth."

Fortunately, while pizza burn hurts, it seldom does serious harm. Your reflexes cue you to stop eating the offending slice almost immediately, so it's not in contact with the mouth tissue long enough to cause lasting damage, says Howard S. Glazer, D.D.S., a dentist in Fort Lee, New Jersey, and past president of the Academy of General Dentistry.

Putting Out the Fire

A pizza burn will heal on its own, usually within 7 to 10 days. "Of all of the parts of the body, the mouth has greatest healing potential," points out Kenneth M. Hargreaves, D.D.S., Ph.D., associate professor in the divisions of endodontics and pharmacology at the University of Minnesota Medical School in Minneapolis. "Almost all of the cells on the surface of the mouth turn over every few days."

So when it comes to treating a pizza burn, your best bet may be to simply let nature take its course. If you want to do something to ease your discomfort in the meantime, try the following tips.

Get wet. "You might get some relief from rinsing your mouth," says Jay W. Friedman, D.D.S., a dental consultant in Los Angeles and

When to See the Dentist

A pizza burn seldom requires medical attention. But see your dentist as soon as possible if you notice swelling in the area of the burn or if the burn does not heal in 7 to 10 days.

author of *Complete Guide to Dental Health*. It doesn't matter if you use warm or cold water, he adds—just go with whichever feels better.

Take a pill for the pain. If you want to try an over-the-counter pain reliever, experts say that just about any nonsteroidal anti-inflammatory drug (NSAID) such as ibuprofen or naproxen (Aleve) will do. But forget the old wives' tale about putting aspirin directly on the injured area to help it heal; it could make matters even worse. "Aspirin is a highly caustic chemical," cautions Dr. Friedman. "It's irritating to the tissue and could cause a fairly serious acid burn."

Numb it. "You can purchase over-the-counter ointments that contain benzocaine (such as Zilactin)," says Dr. Glazer. "Benzocaine is a numbing agent that will help soothe the area."

For something a little stronger, talk to your dentist about using a prescription-strength topical medication.

Don't get irritated. When you're nursing a pizza burn, be careful of what you eat and drink. Try to stick with foods on the mild side, both in temperature and in flavor. And stay away from foods that are spicy or that contain citric acid, such as orange juice, tomato juice, and even highly acidic soft drinks such as colas, says Dr. Price.

If you absolutely must drink an acidic juice, mix it with a little water first. "Diluting the juice reduces the acidic concentration, so it won't burn when you drink it," explains Lawrence Wolinsky, D.M.D., Ph.D., professor of oral biology at the University of California, Los Angeles, School of Dentistry.

Banish the butts. Smoking will just irritate the burn and slow the healing process. So now you have yet another good reason to quit.

Postoperative Pain

You had so much on your mind before your surgery that you really didn't give too much thought to how you were going to feel afterward. Well, hindsight is 20/20, as they say. A long recuperation has left you achy, miserable, and wishing you had been better prepared for the pain.

Well, don't be too hard on yourself. After all, you had every reason to believe that surgery would make you feel better, not worse. That's probably what persuaded you to go through with it in the first place.

And really, it's not at all uncommon for people to say that they had less pain before surgery than they do after. With time they feel better—and you will, too. What's more, "the techniques available today can greatly minimize pain," according to James C. Erickson, M.D., professor of anesthesiology at Northwestern University Medical School in Chicago. "With some procedures, there doesn't have to be any pain at all."

The severity of your postoperative pain depends on a number of factors, including the nature of your surgery, your physical and mental state, your previous experience with pain, and whether you develop any complications. Of course, the quality of the postoperative care you receive is important, too.

On the Road to Recovery

How you take care of yourself after your surgery can make all the difference in how quickly you heal. The right actions and the right attitude can get you back on your feet in no time. Here is what the experts advise for a speedy, pain-free recovery.

When to See the Doctor

"If you're having a significant amount of pain after surgery, speak up about it," urges Michael Ferrante, M.D., director of the program for cancer pain and symptom management at the University of Pennsylvania Medical Center in Philadelphia. "It may not be possible to eliminate the pain entirely, but it can be made more tolerable."

You should consult your physician if your pain gets worse over the course of a day or two, according to Lee Swanstrom, M.D., associate clinical professor in the department of surgery at Oregon Health Sciences University in Portland. Other symptoms to watch for include fever, chills, and redness around the incision—all possible indicators of an infection.

Also let your doctor know if you experience significant side effects from any pain medication that you may have been prescribed.

Ease the ache with ice. Ice is a good local anesthetic and can help reduce pain around your incision during the first 24 hours after surgery, according to Lee Swanstrom, M.D., associate clinical professor in the department of surgery at Oregon Health Sciences University in Portland. He suggests putting crushed ice in a plastic bag, wrapping the bag in a towel, then laying the pack over your incision for as long as you are comfortable.

"Don't use this treatment after the first 24 hours, though," he says. "It can delay wound healing." For the same reason, you should never put anything wet directly on a fresh incision.

Add some heat. After the first 24 hours, trade in your ice bag for a heating pad or hot-water bottle, Dr. Swanstrom suggests. "Heat keeps the muscles around the incision from becoming stiff," he explains. Don't make the pad or bottle too hot, though—just around 100°F. "And be careful not to fall asleep on it," he adds.

Get active as soon as possible. "It's wise to rest for the first day or two after surgery," Dr. Erickson says. "But then you should get up and do some easy walking and gentle exercise. If you stay in bed much longer than that, you'll have a lot more pain when you finally start moving around." Remaining inactive for an extended period of time also increases your risk of postoperative complications.

Lift your spirits. When you're recuperating from surgery, attitude counts, Dr. Swanstrom says. "Try to focus on the fact that every day you feel a little bit better," he urges.

Of course, there may be times when you have more pain than you did the day before. "If you have an off-day, it's usually because you've overdone it," he says. "So ease up a bit—but also look at the overall trend toward improvement."

Medicate when necessary. If your doctor prescribed a painkiller before you left the hospital, take it only when you need to, Dr. Swanstrom says. "If you overuse the medication, you may experience side effects that can actually increase your pain," he explains. "For example, some drugs cause constipation—and when you have just had surgery, you don't want to be straining to move your bowels."

Time it right. While you don't want to overdo it with painkillers, you also don't want to put off taking them until you are doubled over in pain. "If you take your medication when the pain first starts, you may need only one pill," Dr. Swanstrom says. "But if you let your pain get really bad, you may have to take three pills—and you'll still be uncomfortable. It will take an hour or so for the drug to reach its full effectiveness." So when, exactly, should you take your medicine? "When you start noticing an ache or an unpleasant feeling," he advises.

Don't go cold turkey. If you are taking prescription narcotics for your pain, discontinue them as soon as you're able, Dr. Swanstrom says. But don't abruptly stop taking medication altogether, he cautions. Instead, switch to a nonsteroidal anti-inflammatory drug (NSAID) such as ibuprofen for a period of time.

Make a point of trying acupuncture. "Studies have shown that acupuncture can reduce your need for medication," says Felice Dunas, Ph.D., a licensed acupuncturist and a doctor of clinical Chinese medicine in private practice in Topanga, California. "You can take smaller doses for a shorter period of time." Acupuncture also helps clear your body of anesthesia, so you feel better sooner, she says.

Most states have licensing procedures for acupuncturists. Make sure that you choose someone with the proper credentials.

Razor Burn

Every morning, men throughout the world head off to their jobs with tiny shreds of tissue stuck to their cheeks and chins. As they pass each other on the streets, stand side by side on assembly lines, and sit around conference tables, they exchange brief but meaningful glances, as if they were members of some sacred brotherhood. "I know what you're going through," their eyes seem to say. "I feel your pain."

Indeed, razor burn leaves few men unscathed. And those tiny cuts and abrasions inflicted by a menacing blade can be murder on sensitive skin.

But razor burn isn't exclusively a male malady. Women suffer, too. The skin of the legs and underarms is just as vulnerable as the stubbly cheeks of a just-awakened man.

Relief from the Razor's Edge

If you have had previous bouts with razor burn, you may already know about the styptic pencil. Available in drugstores, it is renowned for its ability to stem the flow of blood from those nasty nicks.

But there are other steps you can take to relieve the pain of razor burn—and, even better, to protect your tender skin from future run-ins with a wayward blade. Here is what the experts recommend.

Put on the pressure. If you nick your skin, press directly on the cut with a piece of gauze or a clean cloth, advises Joseph A. Witkowski, M.D., clinical professor of dermatology at the University of Pennsylvania School of Medicine in Philadelphia. Apply steady pressure for 10 to 15 minutes. "And don't peek," Dr. Witkowski cautions. "Every time you peek, you dislodge a clot, making the cut bleed again."

When to See the Doctor

For the most part, razor burn is a minor problem that will heal with proper self-care. But if it happens every time you shave, you may want to see your doctor, says Jerome Z. Litt, M.D., assistant clinical professor of dermatology at Case Western Reserve University School of Medicine in Cleveland.

You should also seek medical attention if your skin becomes infected and crusty or if it is persistently red and scaly, says David Margolis, M.D., assistant professor of dermatology at the University of Pennsylvania Medical Center in Philadelphia. The reason is that razor burn can mimic the symptoms of other skin conditions, such as psoriasis, which require very specific treatments.

Add a dab of ointment. "If the nick is bad, apply antibiotic ointment to prevent infection," advises Jerome Z. Litt, M.D., assistant clinical professor of dermatology at Case Western Reserve University School of Medicine in Cleveland.

Choose the right tool. You should use a new, clean blade for every shave, Dr. Litt says. And if you're using double-track blades, you may want to consider switching to the single-track type. "The advent of double-track blades has produced more cases of razor burn," he contends. "They create irritation and sometimes follicle problems." He recommends Bic's Original or Sensitive Shaver single-track disposable blades instead.

Get steamed. Men should wait until after their showers to shave, Dr. Litt says. The hot steam softens the whiskers, so the blade doesn't yank and pull so much.

Lather up. Shaving cream is a must for men and women alike. "It keeps moisture in the hair follicles and makes the shave smoother," Dr. Litt says.

Just make sure that you're not allergic to the product you're using, cautions David Margolis, M.D., assistant professor of dermatology at the University of Pennsylvania Medical Center in Philadelphia. "If you're sensitive to any of the ingredients, the shaving cream will make your skin red when you use it," he explains. To find out if you are allergic, put a little shaving cream on your arm and cover it with a bandage. Leave it on until the next day, then check for irritation. "If you are allergic, try a different brand—maybe one for sensitive skin or without fragrance," he says.

Check out a gel. You may want to switch from a cream to one of the highly lubricating gels on the market, Dr. Margolis says. "Generally, gel is more lubricating than foam," he notes.

Don't go against the grain. You can reduce your odds of razor burn by shaving in the same direction as your hair growth. "Don't use upward strokes on the cheeks or legs, and don't shave from side to side," Dr. Litt advises. You don't get quite as close a shave this way, but it trains the hairs to grow straight.

Follow directions. The natural growth of a beard may vary from one part of the face to another, Dr. Margolis says. "The hairs may not point in the same direction," he notes. "Let your beard grow for a few days and watch the patterns as the hairs come in."

Don't get too close. "If you try to shave very close—the way television commercials tell you to do—you'll only irritate your skin," says Dr. Margolis. His two rules of thumb: Never stretch your skin while you shave, and don't apply too much pressure with your razor.

This is especially good advice for African-Americans, says Dr. Litt. "A black person's hair grows out in a curl," he explains. "If it's shaved too close, it will grow right back into the skin. This can lead to a follicle infection."

Multiply your moisturizing. Lotions and creams make just-shaved skin feel better. "The best moisturizer is petroleum jelly," says Dr. Margolis. "But if you don't find it cosmetically pleasing, use something bland and not highly scented." Apply it three or four times a day, he adds.

Repetitive Strain Injury

It has been called a modern-day epidemic, and for good reason. Repetitive strain injury accounts for more than half of all occupational illnesses and an estimated $100 billion in lost work time. It can happen to assembly-line workers and competitive athletes, electricians and artists. Anyone who performs the same motion over and over again for long periods of time is a candidate for this condition.

The "strain" part of repetitive strain injury comes from the muscles and tendons that become inflamed as the result of overuse. It most often affects the hands, wrists, elbows, shoulders, and neck.

What makes repetitive strain injury so prevalent these days is the explosion in computer use. People pound away on their keyboards for hours at a time without taking a break, notes Emil Pascarelli, M.D., professor of clinical medicine and a repetitive strain injury specialist at Columbia–Presbyterian Medical Center in New York City. This overuse can set the stage for a host of problems—including perhaps the best-known repetitive strain injury, carpal tunnel syndrome. (For a more detailed discussion of this condition, see the chapter on page 51.)

Rule Out a Repeat Performance

Treatment for repetitive strain injury varies, depending on the body part involved and the severity of the pain. But experts say that there are some basic strategies that anyone can follow to avoid aggravating the condition—even if he has carpal tunnel syndrome. Here's what they recommend.

Do something different. If your job allows it, "break the monotony of repetitive tasks by moving around," suggests Joel Press, M.D., associate professor of clinical physical medicine and rehabilitation at Northwestern University Medical School in Chicago. "Set an alarm to ring every 30 to 45 minutes to remind you."

Perfect your posture. Be aware of how your body is positioned while you perform a repetitive task, advises Dr. Press. "If your job requires you to stand, for example, make sure you're upright, not hunched over the whole time."

Get lined up. If you use a computer, check the placement of your screen and keyboard. "They should be in front of you rather than off to the side, which forces you to twist your body," says Dr. Press.

Check the height. The computer screen should be visible without any neck strain. "Your eyes should gaze slightly downward—not up or way down," Dr. Press advises.

Please be seated—properly. The height of your chair is also important. "Your feet should be flat on the ground, and your thighs should be parallel to the ground," Dr. Press says.

Check your keyboard technique. "When you type, your forearms should be parallel to the floor, and your wrists should be in a neutral (straight) position," says Dr. Pascarelli. "You should use your whole arm to move your hand over the keyboard rather than stretching your fingers to reach the keys."

Also use light keystrokes and avoid leaning on the arms of the chair with your elbows while you type, Dr. Pascarelli says.

Pick up the phone. You're almost guaranteed a repetitive strain injury if you always tuck the telephone receiver between your shoulder and your ear. "If you're on the phone for more than 20 minutes at a time, you should use a headset or a speakerphone instead," says Dr. Press.

Hold your head up. "The head is a large mass atop a small pedestal," observes Leon Robb, M.D., director of the Robb Pain Management Group in Los Angeles. "If you keep it in one position for a long period of time—for example, flexing it forward while you read— you strain your neck muscles and put pressure on the nerves at the

When to See the Doctor

Y ou can be fairly certain that you have a repetitive strain injury if your symptoms subside when you stop the activity
that's causing them, says Joel Press, M.D., associate professor of
clinical physical medicine and rehabilitation at Northwestern University Medical School in Chicago. If pain persists, you should
see your doctor, he advises.

Also seek medical attention if you notice any of the fol-
lowing symptoms, says Leon Robb, M.D., director of the Robb
Pain Management Group in Los Angeles.
- Pain that radiates to other parts of your body
- Severe pain when you lie down (especially if it disrupts your
  sleep)
- Numbness or tingling, along with pain
- Clumsiness that you can't control, even when you fully con-
  centrate on what you're doing

back of your neck." The resulting pain can radiate into your head, face,
and arms, he adds.

Shrug off the pain. Shoulder shrugs can help protect your
neck from repetitive strain injury, according to Dr. Robb. Simply shrug
your shoulders, hold for 2 to 3 seconds, then relax. Do five to six repetitions every 2 to 3 hours. You may want to hold very light weights (no
more than 1 pound) in your hands to build up your upper back muscles.

Arm yourself against harm. Your hands, wrists, and arms
are the body parts most at risk for repetitive strain injury. To increase
their strength and flexibility, Dr. Pascarelli recommends the following
exercises.
1. Hold your left arm straight in front of you at shoulder level.
   (Maintain this position for all of the exercises.)
2. Place your right hand over the knuckles of your left hand and
   gently press downward, so the fingers of your left hand are

pointing straight down and the palm is facing you. Hold for a count of 10. Repeat three times.

3. Make a fist with your left hand. Place your right hand over the knuckles of your left hand and gently press your fist downward. Hold for a count of 10. Repeat three times.

4. Position your left hand so that your palm is facing up. Then bend your wrist backward as far as you can so that your fingers are pointing toward the floor. Place your right hand on the palm side of your left hand, over the knuckle joints, and gently pull your left hand back toward your body. Hold for a count of 10, then relax. Repeat three times.

5. Position your left hand so that your fingers are pointing upward and your palm is facing away from you, as though you were signaling someone to stop. Place your right hand on the palm side of your left hand, over the knuckle joints, and carefully press your left hand back toward you. Hold for a count of 10. Repeat three times.

6. Repeat the sequence with your right hand.

Dr. Pascarelli suggests repeating the entire series three to five times with each hand.

Sciatica

I t's a pain in the butt—quite literally. It can also be a pain in the hip, the thigh, the lower leg, or even the foot. In fact, the condition known as sciatica can send pain shooting anywhere in your lower body.

What's causing all the commotion is the sciatic nerve, which is not one but a group of nerves bound together in a single sheath. The sciatic nerve runs from your lower back down each leg all the way to the foot. When it is injured, inflamed, or irritated, it can produce pain at any point—or every point—along its route.

The most common cause of sciatica is a herniated disk. "Disks separate the vertebrae in your spine," explains Garth Russell, M.D., clinical professor of orthopedics at the University of Missouri—Columbia School of Medicine and senior surgeon at the Columbia Spine Center, both in Columbia. "Each one has a fluid center surrounded by stretchable fibrous tissue. When a disk becomes herniated, the tissue balloons out, like a bulge on a tire." Depending on the disk's location, it can put pressure directly on the sciatic nerve, which doesn't take too kindly to the intrusion. The result is excruciating pain.

On rare occasions, sciatica can result from other health problems. Some are serious, such as diabetes, blood clots, and tumors. But others are minor: You can even get sciatic pain from sitting too long in an awkward position. So have your pain checked out before you proceed with self-care.

You Have Some Nerve!

Sciatica usually subsides in a matter of days with proper self-care. To help speed the healing process—and to protect yourself from another bout of sciatic pain—give these strategies a try.

Write your own prescription. Nonsteroidal anti-inflammatory drugs (NSAIDs) such as ibuprofen remain the treatment of choice for sciatica, according to Dr. Russell. "They can reduce any nerve inflammation caused by the pressure of a herniated disk," he explains. These medications won't cure your pain, but they will make it more tolerable.

Lighten your load. "Limit your physical activity," Dr. Russell advises. "Avoid standing, lifting, and sitting for long periods of time. Let pain be your guide: Do what doesn't hurt, and don't do what does hurt."

Get up and at 'em. Don't lay off for too long, though. "You shouldn't be on your back for more than a week," Dr. Russell says. "It's important to start moving around as quickly as possible."

Take a seat the right way. When you do have to sit, make sure that your posture doesn't make your sciatica worse, says Stella Shigenaka, a physical therapist at the Institute of Progressive Physical Therapy in Los Angeles. "Your knees and hips should be bent at about 90-degree angles," she advises. "Your weight should be on the ischium tuberosity—the sitting bones—and not on the tailbone."

Give yourself a break. Don't sit for more than 40 minutes at a stretch, Shigenaka advises. Plan frequent breaks, allowing yourself time to get up and move around.

Give your legs a lift. Try to keep pressure off the lumbar region of your spine, from which most sciatic pain radiates, says Scott Haldeman, M.D., D.C., Ph.D., associate clinical professor of neurology at the University of California, Irvine. He suggests lying on your back with your lower legs resting on a chair or a low table (such as a coffee table). Your knees and hips should be bent at about 90-degree angles. Do this as needed for relief, he says.

Flex your pelvis. Pelvic tilts allow you to gently move the lumbar region of your spine, increasing circulation in the area, Dr. Haldeman says. His instructions: Lie on your back with your feet on the floor and your knees bent. Tilt your pelvis so that your back flat-

When to See the Doctor

E xperts say that it's a good idea to consult your doctor when sciatica first sets in. Since many things can cause sciatica—some of them quite serious—you need a doctor to determine what's behind your pain.

Once you have a diagnosis, alert your doctor immediately if you experience any of the following symptoms, according to Scott Haldeman, M.D., D.C., Ph.D., associate clinical professor of neurology at the University of California, Irvine.

- Paralysis in the affected leg
- Marked loss of sensation or coordination in the affected leg
- Loss of bowel or bladder function
- Pain that persists for more than a month, especially if it gets progressively worse

tens against the ground, then lift it up. Hold for 5 seconds and relax. Continue tilting and lifting and relaxing five to six times every hour when sciatica flares up.

Go for yoga. Practicing certain yoga exercises can help ease sciatic pain, according to Mary Pullig Schatz, M.D., a pathologist and yoga instructor in Nashville and author of *Back Care Basics*. Here are the two she recommends.

- Lie on your back with your calves resting on the seat of a chair. Your hips and knees should be bent at about 90-degree angles. Cross your arms over your chest and place your hands on your shoulders, not on your neck. Inhale, then begin a long, slow exhalation. During the exhalation, tilt your pelvis so that your lower back moves to the floor as you flatten your abdomen. Raise your shoulders 6 to 10 inches off the ground. Lower your right shoulder to touch the floor, then raise it back up. Inhale as you lower your trunk to the floor. Repeat, this time lowering and raising your left shoulder instead. Do this five to six times per side.

• Lie on your back with a rolled-up towel behind your neck for support and a folded towel under your head. Place your arms at your sides, palms facing up. Bend both knees and together draw them toward your chest as you exhale. Then while you inhale, slowly and gently lower one knee toward the floor on one side of your body. Rest it there for 5 to 6 seconds. On the exhalation, slowly lift your knee back to the starting position. Repeat on the other side, then repeat the entire sequence three to five times.
Note: This exercise is not suitable for women in the second half of pregnancy.

Pamper your piriformis. Sometimes sciatica results from a tight piriformis muscle, according to Dr. Schatz. This muscle extends from the side of the sacrum (a triangular bone formed by five fused vertebrae in the lower portion of the spine) to the top of the thighbone at the hip joint. Along the way it passes over the sciatic nerve.

Dr. Schatz recommends this exercise to gently stretch the pir iformis so it lengthens over time: Sit on the corner of a neatly folded blanket that is 4 to 6 inches high, with your knees bent and your feet flat on the floor in front of you. Slide your right foot under your left knee, positioning it next to your left buttock. Then place your left foot on the floor next to the outside of your right thigh. You should feel your weight resting equally on both sitting bones. Allow your spine to lengthen upward as you gently lift your breastbone. Stabilize your trunk by holding your left knee with both hands. Repeat the exercise two to four times on each side, holding the pose for 20 seconds at first and gradually building up to a few minutes. Over time, you may want to decrease the thickness of the blanket until you can sit on the floor.

"It is of utmost importance that the pose be adjusted so that you feel a minimum amount of discomfort," Dr. Schatz advises. "If the muscle is stretched too vigorously, the pain will become unbearable and the muscle will go into spasm, making your sciatica even worse."

Don't get crossed. "You tend to cross the same leg all the time," Shigenaka says. "That means you're always sitting on the same buttock, which puts a lot of pressure on the sciatic nerve on that side."

Ideally, you shouldn't cross your legs at all. But if you must, at least try to switch sides from time to time.

Lose your wallet. Men often get sciatica from sitting on a bulky wallet. "Move your wallet to a side pocket, or keep it in your jacket," Shigenaka suggests. "If you're driving, put it on the seat or in your briefcase."

Adjust your seat. "Most people position the car seat too far back when they drive," Shigenaka says. "You put a lot of strain on your back when you have to stretch to reach the pedals. You should be able to press the gas pedal just by flexing your ankle. Your hips should be at about a 90-degree angle, and your back should be in neutral— not bent, not perfectly straight, but comfortable."

Shingles

S ure, you've fantasized about reliving your youth. But this most definitely is not what you had in mind. It seems the virus that gave you chicken pox decades ago has decided to pay a return visit. Only this time around, it has produced shingles (also known as herpes zoster)—a painful rash that eventually erupts into clusters of pus-filled blisters.

Truth be known, the chicken pox virus has been loitering around in certain nerve cells of your body since you first picked it up from one of your kindergarten classmates. Scientists can't yet explain what causes it to become active after lying dormant for so long. Among the suspected triggers are stress, injury, or a temporary weakness in the immune system. Age appears to be a factor, too: Shingles is most common in people over age 50.

Shingles' trademark rash typically appears on one side of the body, following the path of the affected nerve from the midline of the chest to the midline of the back. Sometimes it spreads to the face as well. If this happens to you, you should see your doctor right away: If the eyes become involved, you could end up with permanent vision damage.

In older people shingles sometimes leads to a condition known as postherpetic neuralgia. The pain persists for months or even years after the rash disappears.

Nailing Down the Pain

Not everyone who had chicken pox as a child develops shingles as an adult. If you're one of the unlucky ones, you should head for your doctor at the first sign of an outbreak, advises Timothy Berger,

What to Do When the Pain Won't Stop

For some people, the pain of shingles lingers long after the actual rash disappears. This condition, called postherpetic neuralgia, can go on for months or even years.

The prescription drug acyclovir (Zovirax) can reduce the duration and intensity of pain, but often more is required. Here's what the experts recommend to help stop the hurting.

Apply ice. Rubbing ice on the affected area can provide temporary relief, says Leon Robb, M.D., director of the Robb Pain Management Group in Los Angeles. Heat, however, can do more harm than good, he cautions.

Zap it with Zostrix. Zostrix is an ointment that contains capsaicin, the substance that makes hot peppers hot. It acts on nerve endings to reduce the sensation of pain, explains Clay J. Cockerell, M.D., associate professor of dermatology and pathology at the University of Texas Southwestern Medical Center at Dallas. He suggests that you apply the ointment to the affected area every 4 hours around the clock. Just be sure your blisters have healed before using this treatment, he says.

Learn to relax. A relaxation technique such as meditation or visualization can help you manage your pain, says Bradley Galer, M.D., assistant professor of neurology and anesthesiology at the University of Washington School of Medicine in Seattle.

Know your options. A number of prescription medications have proved effective in treating postherpetic neuralgia, says Dr. Galer. Among the most promising are tricyclic antidepressants, antiseizure drugs such as hydantoin and carbamazepine, and narcotics. A new formulation of lidocaine has also shown potential. "It's a medicated gel in a patch," Dr. Galer explains. "It can be placed right over the painful region so it's absorbed through the skin."

None of these drugs will work for everyone, Dr. Galer notes. You need to talk to your doctor about which one may be right for you.

M.D., associate clinical professor of dermatology at the University of California, San Francisco, School of Medicine. Your doctor will most likely give you a prescription for acyclovir (Zovirax), which will help reduce not only the duration of the rash but also the duration of the pain, he says.

To help ease your discomfort while you're on the mend, give these tips a try.

Apply a cooling compress. "Soak some gauze or a washcloth in cool, clean water or a saline solution and put it directly on the blisters," suggests Clay J. Cockerell, M.D., associate professor of dermatology and pathology at the University of Texas Southwestern Medical Center at Dallas. The compress will dry out the blisters and speed the healing process, he explains. It will also help prevent secondary bacterial infection, which can lead to ulceration and scarring.

Pick a painkiller. Acetaminophen and nonsteroidal anti-inflammatory drugs (NSAIDs) such as aspirin and ibuprofen can relieve shingles pain, Dr. Cockerell says. "If an over-the-counter pain reliever doesn't help, your doctor may prescribe a stronger medication such as codeine," he adds.

Strike gold with silver. Many doctors are recommending colloidal silver for shingles because it may have some antiviral and antibacterial action, says Cynthia M. Watson, M.D., a family practitioner in private practice in Santa Monica, California. "When it's applied directly to the blisters, they seem to dry up in a matter of days." Colloidal silver can be purchased in health food stores.

Wash up. Clean the affected area with soap and water, then apply 3 percent hydrogen peroxide, advises Leon Robb, M.D., director of the Robb Pain Management Group in Los Angeles. Doing so will help prevent the sores from becoming infected.

Nip infection in the bud. If you notice any signs of infection such as redness, swelling, fever, pain, or pus discharge, treat the blisters immediately with an iodine preparation (such as Betadine), Dr. Robb suggests. These products are available over the counter.

When to See the Doctor

You should seek medical attention at the first sign of a shingles outbreak, says Clay J. Cockerell, M.D., associate professor of dermatology and pathology at the University of Texas Southwestern Medical Center at Dallas. "If you catch shingles early enough, you can cure it fairly quickly," he says. "If you act too late—after five days or so—treatment won't be nearly as effective."

It's especially important to see your doctor if shingles spreads to your face. You want to make sure that it doesn't affect your eyes. If that happens, it could damage your vision permanently, Dr. Cockerell says.

Choose lighter attire. The skin is extra sensitive during a shingles outbreak. "The gentlest touch can be perceived as pain," Dr. Cockerell notes. For this reason, he recommends wearing light, loose-fitting clothes—"nothing that's restrictive or that rubs the skin."

Go under wraps. You can also protect the affected area by wrapping it with an elastic bandage, Dr. Cockerell says. This will prevent anything from touching or rubbing against the blistered skin. "Just be sure the bandage is tight," he cautions. "If it's loose, it will irritate the blisters." Be sure to place a nonadhesive gauze pad over the blisters before wrapping.

If you can't wrap the affected area, Dr. Cockerell suggests coating gauze with petroleum jelly, then taping it over the blisters.

Don't share your pain. "Shingles is less infectious than chicken pox because the virus is not airborne," Dr. Cockerell explains. "Still, the virus can be transmitted by direct contact."

When you have shingles, you should avoid contact with anyone who has not had chicken pox. "Wait until the blisters are crusted over, which usually takes four or five days," Dr. Cockerell says. If you do happen to infect someone, though, the person will develop chicken pox rather than shingles.

Shinsplints

D on't let their name fool you. Shinsplints are not therapeutic devices for aching lower legs. On the contrary, they inflict pain rather than relieving it.

For a more accurate description of this condition, you might want to think in terms of its medical moniker: anterior compartment syndrome. When you have shinsplints, the tissues that surround muscles in the shin region become irritated, producing razor-sharp pain midway down the outside of the tibia, or shinbone.

Invariably, shinsplints are the result of overuse. They are quite common among runners, whose shins take a pounding from workouts on hard surfaces. But you can just as easily get them from a less jarring activity such as dancing or even walking, especially when you do it longer or harder than your muscles are accustomed to.

Say "Sayonara" to Sore Shins

As much as shinsplints hurt, they're seldom serious. Even better, they respond quite well to self-care. Here is what the experts advise to relieve pain fast.

Cut it out. The first course of action in treating shinsplints may also be the toughest for some people: You must ease up on the activity that is causing your pain.

"If you have shinsplints and you maintain the same level of activity, your symptoms won't go away," says Enyi Okereke, M.D., chief of foot and ankle surgery at the University of Pennsylvania Medical Center in Philadelphia. "You want to cut back to the point where you don't have symptoms anymore." You may even have to stop running or walking for a few days.

Run Away from Pain

O f all the activities that can do your shins in, running exacts the heaviest toll. Experts offer these tips to make the miles more shin-friendly for runners.

If the shoe doesn't fit, replace it. "Shoes are like tires," says Stella Shigenaka, a physical therapist at the Institute of Progressive Physical Therapy in Los Angeles. "They're made to last only so many miles, and you have to change them every so often. If they no longer provide shock absorption, you're more prone to shinsplints."

Most running shoes are built for 200 to 300 miles of wear and tear, adds Glenn Gastwirth, D.P.M., deputy executive director of the American Podiatric Medical Association. "That may sound like a lot," he says. "But if you run 10 miles a week, you need a new pair of shoes every 30 weeks."

Tie one on. "Laces are better than Velcro for adjusting a shoe's support and accommodating the changes in your foot as it swells during a workout," explains Enyi Okereke, M.D., chief of foot and ankle surgery at the University of Pennsylvania Medical Center in Philadelphia.

Choose a new location. "The harder the surface you run on, the more prone you are to shinsplints," says Dr. Okereke. "Everything else being equal, a sidewalk or artificial turf is worse than sand or natural turf."

Shorten your stride. "A too-long stride can contribute to shinsplints," Dr. Gastwirth says. "But don't change it too much—running should not be unnatural."

Gain on pain with bromelain. "Bromelain, an enzyme found in pineapple and papaya, works well for inflammatory conditions like shinsplints," says Cynthia M. Watson, M.D., a family practitioner in private practice in Santa Monica, California. You can buy bromelain in pill form in health food stores.

Stay cool. Ice is a good therapy for the first few days that you have pain, says William S. Case, president of Case Physical Therapy in Houston. He suggests this treatment: Fill a paper cup with water and freeze it. Then peel back the top inch or so of the cup to expose the ice. Rub the ice on the painful site for 15 minutes. Do this twice a day.

Then make it hot. After the third day, switch from ice to heat, Case says. "Apply moist heat—a bath, a shower, or a moist heating pad will do—for 15 minutes once or twice a day," he advises.

If you opt for a heating pad, first rub vinegar on your sore shin and then cover the area with plastic, suggests Arthur H. Brownstein, M.D., a physician in Princeville, Hawaii, and clinical instructor of medicine at the University of Hawaii School of Medicine in Manoa. Then place the heating pad over top.

Mend with massage. Massage can increase blood flow to the painful area, which facilitates healing, says Stella Shigenaka, a physical therapist at the Institute of Progressive Physical Therapy in Los Angeles. "The form that's best for shinsplints is called cross-friction massage. It can be painful, though, so it's best to have it done by a physical therapist or massage therapist."

Adapt your workout. While you don't want to do anything to aggravate your shinsplints, that doesn't mean you should become a couch potato. "A stationary bicycle provides a good alternative workout," Case says. "Start with 5- to 10-minute sessions, two or three times a day, working up to 20-minute sessions." Be sure the cycle is set at minimum tension, he adds.

Shigenaka offers another option: running in a swimming pool. Because of the water's buoyancy, your shins are protected from pounding and shock, she explains.

Add some support. You may develop shinsplints if you overpronate (meaning you walk on the inner margins of your feet) or if you have fallen arches, says Thomas Rizzo, Jr., M.D., a physiatrist in the department of physical medicine and rehabilitation at the Mayo Clinic in Jacksonville, Florida. If that's the case, over-the-counter shoe inserts can help.

When to See the Doctor

In most cases the pain of shinsplints disappears when you give your legs some time off. But you should see your doctor if your pain lasts longer than two weeks or if you're having trouble bearing weight on the affected leg, says Enyi Okereke, M.D., chief of foot and ankle surgery at the University of Pennsylvania Medical Center in Philadelphia. "These symptoms could indicate that something more serious is going on, such as a stress fracture."

Get up and running—gradually. Once the pain subsides, you'll feel that you can resume your normal level of activity. But take it slow at first. "If you're used to running a certain number of miles, for example, start at about two-thirds the distance," Dr. Okereke suggests. "If you don't notice any symptoms, then continue to add mileage over the course of two weeks."

Build your best defense. Experts agree that strengthening the lower leg muscles is the best way to prevent shinsplints from happening again. You can condition these muscles with the following two exercises.

- Stand with both knees straight, holding on to a table or a chair for support. Rise up on your toes and hold for 5 seconds, then lower your heels to the floor. Start with 10 repetitions and gradually work up to 30. Do the exercise two or three times a day.
- Stand facing a wall. Place your hands on the wall and lean toward it, with one leg forward and one leg back. Keep your back straight and your feet flat on the floor. You should feel a gentle stretch in the calf muscles of the back leg. Hold for 20 seconds to 3 minutes, then switch legs. Repeat twice a day.

Shoulder Pain

You began your Saturday with 18 holes of golf, then followed up with an afternoon of trimming hedges, pulling weeds, and planting flowers. Now it's bedtime, and you can barely raise your arm to brush your hair. It's as if your shoulder were saying, "Enough is enough!"

It has every reason to balk. After all, your shoulders work very hard over the course of a day. They're involved in numerous routine tasks, from turning doorknobs to writing notes.

Among all the joints in your body, your shoulders are perhaps the most versatile. They combine with a variety of tendons and muscles to give your arms their broad range of motion.

But there's a price to be paid for this mobility: The shoulder's construction just begs for trouble. Basically, the rounded end of one bone rests against a shallow cavity in another bone, like a golf ball sitting on a tee. This makes the joint very unstable, vulnerable to injury and other problems. Sprains, strains, and dislocations are common, as are arthritis, bursitis, and tendinitis. (For more information about arthritis and bursitis, see the respective chapters on pages 7 and 36.)

All the Right Moves

So you feel as though you've been carrying the weight of the world on your shoulders—literally. The good news is that you don't have to just grin and bear the burden of pain. Here is what the experts suggest for fast relief.

Stop what you're doing. If a particular activity has aggravated your shoulder, then give it up or at least cut back for the time being, experts say. "And avoid any movement that can make your pain

When to See the Doctor

Any injury to your shoulder requires immediate medical attention, especially if it is accompanied by loss of arm movement or if your shoulder feels as though it's slipping out of place, says David Altchek, M.D., assistant professor of orthopedic surgery at Cornell University Medical College in New York City and team physician for the New York Mets. You should also see your doctor when:

- You experience extreme pain.
- The pain lasts for more than three weeks.
- You notice any swelling or redness.
- You have a fever or chills along with the pain.

worse—mainly reaching over or behind your head," advises Joel Press, M.D., associate professor of clinical physical medicine and rehabilitation at Northwestern University Medical School in Chicago.

Limit lifting. It's also a good idea to refrain from heavy lifting while your shoulder is sore, says David Altchek, M.D., assistant professor of orthopedic surgery at Cornell University Medical College in New York City and team physician for the New York Mets. His rule of thumb: "Don't hoist anything heavier than a briefcase or a gallon of milk."

Keep moving. While you should take it easy, you don't want to completely immobilize an ailing shoulder, according to Phillip A. Bauman, M.D., clinical instructor in orthopedic surgery at the Columbia University College of Physicians and Surgeons and associate attending physician of orthopedic surgery at St. Luke's/Roosevelt Hospital Center, both in New York City. "The longer you limit your movement, the stiffer you become," he says. "That can lead to more pain, which causes you to limit your movement even more. Eventually, you could end up with frozen shoulder," a condition characterized by severe pain and stiffness.

Make nice with ice. Applying ice for the first few days that your shoulder hurts can help reduce inflammation, Dr. Altchek says. He recommends using a "freezable" gel pack, which you can purchase in a drugstore. Wrap the pack in a thin towel and lay it on top of your shoulder, perhaps wrapping an elastic bandage around it to keep it in place. Leave it on for no more than 20 minutes and reapply it three times a day.

Switch to heat. Once the inflammation subsides, you can begin treating your sore shoulder with heat, Dr. Altchek says. "It can help loosen up your shoulder if you are stiff," he notes. "Just be sure that you use moist heat, like a hot shower, rather than dry heat, like a heating pad."

Up the ante with an anti-inflammatory. Dr. Press recommends taking an over-the-counter nonsteroidal anti-inflammatory drug (NSAID) such as ibuprofen. "If it doesn't help, check with your doctor," he says. "Your doctor could prescribe a stronger dose."

Get back in the swing. Gentle stretching and range-of-motion exercises are important to your shoulder's rehabilitation because they help restore and improve flexibility, says Ed Laskowski, M.D., co-director of the Sportsmedicine Center at the Mayo Clinic in Rochester, Minnesota. Experts recommend the following moves to keep your shoulder loose and limber.

- Move the arm on the same side as your sore shoulder across your chest, toward the opposite shoulder. Then gently pull the arm toward you by placing the opposite hand over the elbow. You should feel the stretch in the back of your shoulder. Hold for at least 15 seconds. Repeat at least three times a day.
- Stand in a corner with your hands above shoulder height on either wall. Lean into the corner with your body, as though you were doing a push-up. Hold for 10 to 15 seconds. Repeat 10 times, twice a day. This exercise stretches your chest muscles, which support your shoulders.
- Lie in bed on your back. Slowly raise the arm on the same side as your sore shoulder above your head so that it rests on a pillow or

the mattress. Hold that position for 10 to 15 seconds, then return your arm to your side. Repeat three times. Do this stretch twice a day—first thing when you get up in the morning and last thing before you go to sleep.

- Bend at your waist and dangle both arms so that they're perpendicular to the floor. Let your arms make slow circles, like a pendulum. You shouldn't really have to move them—allow gravity to do the work. Continue for 1 to 2 minutes. Repeat no more than three times a day.

Test your flexibility. "You should be able to raise your arms overhead, both from the side and from the front," says John Cianca, M.D., assistant professor of physical medicine and rehabilitation at Baylor College of Medicine in Houston. He recommends practicing these movements until you can do them easily. "Also practice reaching up behind your back, as if you were unhooking a bra," he says. "But don't try so hard that you strain yourself."

Move your body right. Whether you're a weekend warrior or a serious athlete, you can avoid a repeat performance of your shoulder injury by having an expert check out your body mechanics, Dr. Press advises. A qualified fitness trainer or coach can spot what you are doing incorrectly—when you swing your tennis racquet or lift a barbell, for example—and teach you proper form and technique.

Side Stitches

A good joke can leave you in stitches. But a side stitch is nothing to laugh about. That familiar stabbing pain in the lower part of the rib cage is far from life threatening. But it comes on so suddenly and is so excruciating that it's guaranteed to stop you in your tracks.

A side stitch occurs when your diaphragm or another muscle in the abdominal region abruptly contracts, usually during vigorous physical activity. The spasm affects your breathing, and you can't meet your body's oxygen demands. You have to take a break from what you're doing and wait for the pain to subside before you can continue.

Experts don't yet know for sure what triggers a side stitch. Among the more common theories are engaging in an activity that is too strenuous for your level of conditioning, breathing improperly, becoming dehydrated, and exercising too soon after a meal.

Give Your Stitch the Slip

A side stitch seldom lasts longer than 10 minutes. And once it's gone, it's gone—you won't feel any aftereffects. None of this matters, though, when a stitch has you in its grip. Then all you can think about is relief.

Here are some things you can do to keep stitches from tying you in knots.

Put on the brakes. "Don't try to work through a side stitch," says Brent S. E. Rich, M.D., staff physician at Arizona Orthopaedic and Sports Medicine Specialists in Phoenix and team physician at Arizona State University in Tempe. "If you're running, for example, slow down to a walk or sit and rest. The stitch will gradually go away."

When to See the Doctor

A side stitch is not serious enough to warrant medical attention. In fact, it would probably disappear by the time you got to your doctor's office. "But if you get a stitch every time you exert yourself, ask your physician to check your hydration and electrolyte status," says Brent S. E. Rich, M.D., staff physician at Arizona Orthopaedic and Sports Medicine Specialists in Phoenix and team physician at Arizona State University in Tempe. (Electrolytes—nutrients such as potassium and sodium—regulate your body's chemical balance.)

Reach for the sky. Once you stop moving, raise your arms overhead, advises John Cianca, M.D., assistant professor of physical medicine and rehabilitation at Baylor College of Medicine in Houston. "This allows your chest to expand and contract more when you breathe," he explains. "It stretches the muscles, too."

Restart gradually. Once the pain subsides, says Dr. Rich, you can resume your activity, but at a lower intensity. "If the stitch returns, stop again," he advises. "It won't escalate into anything serious, but your body won't let you continue."

Watch your breath. Proper breathing technique may help prevent side stitches, says Dr. Cianca. "When you exercise, take longer, deeper breaths," he suggests. "Short, choppy breathing tends to overwork the muscles. It's better to regulate your breathing so you inhale and exhale in rhythm with the movement of your limbs."

Warm up beforehand. Jumping headlong into vigorous exercise is an invitation for a side stitch. "Be sure to warm up enough," says Dr. Cianca. "Stretch, loosen up, rev up your body before you work out."

Don't eat and run. Making demands on your body too soon after you feed it is a definite no-no. "Wait 45 to 60 minutes after eating before you exercise," advises Dr. Rich.

Lighten up. What you eat is just as important as when you eat. "A side stitch is more likely to occur after a heavy meal than after a light one," says Dr. Rich. "So eat something light when you know that you're going to be exercising. And avoid spicy, greasy, and fatty foods—they slow down the digestive process."

He recommends fueling your body with carbohydrate-rich foods such as pasta and bread. "They're easier to digest, and they won't give you a heavy feeling when you exercise," he says.

Drink to your health. "Make sure that you're well-hydrated, especially if you're working out in the heat," says Dr. Rich. "As a rule of thumb, drink 8 to 12 ounces of fluids before you start exercising, then 4 to 8 ounces every 30 to 45 minutes while you're on the move." The best choices for proper hydration are water, fruit juices, and sports drinks (such as Gatorade).

Don't hit the bottle. Drinking and working out don't mix. "Avoid alcohol before exercise," advises Dr. Rich. "It acts as a diuretic and can lead to dehydration."

Sinus Pain

If you have sinus trouble, you may rue the day when your prehistoric ancestors first stood on their own two feet. The tiny passages that connect the sinuses to the nose were perfectly situated for drainage when humankind got around on all fours. But this design doesn't work nearly as well now that we're walking upright.

Your sinuses are lined with a membrane that manufactures the sticky substance known as mucus. When the membrane swells—most likely because of an infection or an allergy—mucus production kicks into overdrive. The combination of inflamed membrane and excess mucus blocks those tiny passages between your sinuses and nose. That's when you feel the pressure build behind your forehead and eyes.

But sinus pain isn't always what it seems. "For example, sometimes patients think that they have a sinus infection when what they really have is a migraine," notes Salah D. Salman, M.D., director of the Sinus Center at the Massachusetts Eye and Ear Infirmary in Boston. Both of these conditions produce a distinct my-head-is-going-to-explode-any-minute-now feeling.

Breathe a Sigh of Relief

For most people decongestants are the treatment of choice for sinus pain. (That may explain why sinus medicines are a $1.5 billion industry in the United States.) "If a blocked nose is your only symptom, an over-the-counter oral decongestant can help," Dr. Salman says. "Be sure to choose a product with an antihistamine if your sinus pain is associated with allergy."

What about localized decongestants such as sprays and drops? "They can be extremely effective, too," Dr. Salman says. "But you

---

Decipher Your Sinus Symptoms

The best way to treat sinus pain is to figure out what's causing it. The following guidelines can help you determine exactly what's bugging you (but see your doctor, just to be sure).

- If your nose drips clear, watery mucus and you have discomfort when you stoop down, a sense of heaviness in the front of your face, and a general feeling of malaise, you probably have a viral infection.
- If, in addition to pain and congestion, your eyes are itchy and red, you probably have an allergy.
- If the mucus is yellow or green, you probably have a bacterial infection. (This requires treatment with antibiotics.)
- If the pain comes and goes in a day or so and you have few or no cold symptoms, you may have a tension (vascular) headache.
- If the pain is more to one side and is accompanied by nausea or vomiting, you may have a migraine.

shouldn't use them for more than three days in a row. They can be habit forming if you use them for too long. And once their medicinal effects wear off, they can produce rebound congestion."

But decongestants are not your only option for dealing with sinus pain. The following strategies can help ease the pressure and keep you breathing easy.

Turn on the steam. A steam inhaler can provide fast relief from sinus pain, according to Guillermo Mendoza, M.D., chief of allergy for Kaiser–Permanente at Vacaville in California. "The device looks like a pilot's mask," he explains. "You put tap water in it and it creates steam. It's relaxing, and it makes you feel better for a few hours." You can purchase a steam inhaler in a drugstore or a medical supply store.

Just add water. "Dryness often sets the stage for a sinus infection," Dr. Salman says. You can keep your sinuses moist by

When to See the Doctor

T here's something to be said for letting nature take its course with a mild sinus infection," says Guillermo Mendoza, M.D., chief of allergy for Kaiser–Permanente at Vacaville in California. "But if the infection doesn't go away in three to five days or if your pain is severe, you should see your doctor." Untreated, a severe sinus infection can lead to bronchitis or asthma. It's also close enough to the eyes and brain to be of some concern.

You should also see your doctor if your sinus pain is accompanied by fever; swollen or red eyes; double vision; or fatigue, lethargy, or sleepiness, says Salah D. Salman, M.D., director of the Sinus Center at the Massachusetts Eye and Ear Infirmary in Boston.

drinking plenty of water every day—at least eight 8-ounce glasses, experts advise. A saltwater solution, administered as either a nasal spray or nose drops, can also help, he notes. You can make your own solution by mixing 2 tablespoons of salt into a glass filled with 8 ounces of warm water. Use this preparation three to four times a day.

Hold your head high. Elevating your head while you sleep promotes sinus drainage, experts say. Prop up your bedposts at the head of your bed on books or bricks and see if it helps.

Clear the air. Anything that irritates the nasal passages is an ally of sinus pain. "Pay attention to air quality," Dr. Mendoza advises. "Avoid smoggy environments, cigarette smoke, and any other pollutants that you're sensitive to." You may also need to stay away from seemingly harmless items such as scented laundry detergents and scented tissues.

Be doubly clean. Use two-ply vacuum cleaner bags, Dr. Mendoza suggests: "They are stronger and less porous than regular bags, so they do not allow dirt and dust to filter through." When that happens, the particles can irritate your nasal passages and cause sinus pain.

Put out that cigarette. Smoking not only irritates your nasal passages but also undermines your natural resistance to infection, experts say. This double whammy is an open invitation to sinus pain.

"C" your way clear. Dr. Mendoza recommends a daily dose of vitamin C as a preventive against sinus pain. "If you are prone to sinus infection or you have a chronic sinus problem, take 1,000 milligrams of timed-release vitamin C a day," he advises.

Don't catch a cold. If you have a chronic sinus problem, a cold will only intensify your symptoms, Dr. Mendoza says. So do what you can to steer clear of cold-causing viruses: Eat a balanced diet, get regular exercise, practice good hygiene (as in lots of hand washing), and stay away from people who have colds.

Sore Throat

For the younger set a sore throat often means a day off from school, a television tuned to the Cartoon Network, and an extra-big bowl of ice cream. It almost makes the suffering seem worthwhile.

Grown-ups, of course, don't have time for such pampering. We go about our daily business, thinking we can tough out the rawness, burning, and scratchiness that make it painful to talk—much less swallow food. But by day's end, the sore throat has left us virtually speechless.

We do tend to think of a sore throat as kid stuff. But the fact is that every year about 40 million adults come down with one. Usually it is a symptom of a viral or bacterial infection. But it can also be instigated by irritants such as stomach acid, tobacco smoke, smog, dry heat, dust, pollen, and other allergens. Overuse is also a factor: You know what happens when you spend an entire evening shouting to your friends over the din of loud music, or you cheer too long and too loud at a football game.

Silence Your Symptoms

A sore throat usually goes away on its own within a few days. But you don't have to suffer in the meantime. Try the following tips to soothe the soreness fast.

Make like Marcel Marceau. "Don't talk if you don't have to," says Oscar Janiger, M.D., associate clinical professor at the University of California, Irvine, School of Medicine and author of *A Different Kind of Healing.* It may seem obvious, yet a lot of folks prolong their pain by not heeding this advice.

In a State of Reflux

We tend to associate sore throat with colds and flu. But in some cases, it's really the stomach that's to blame. "Probably about 25 percent of the population has some degree of gastroesophageal reflux," says Charles N. Ford, M.D., professor and chairman of otolaryngology at the University of Wisconsin Medical School in Madison. "Stomach acid percolates up the esophagus and into the back of the throat, usually while you're asleep and not aware of it. You may wake up with a gravelly voice and discomfort."

If you have a problem with reflux, Dr. Ford recommends taking the following actions.

- Cut down on spicy foods.
- Eat your biggest meal earlier in the day rather than in the evening.
- Take an antacid at bedtime and ½ hour after consuming anything spicy.
- Keep your head elevated while you sleep so that stomach acid stays in your stomach and doesn't head north.

Turn down the volume. If you must talk, then refrain from using your voice in an unnatural way, says Charles N. Ford, M.D., professor and chairman of otolaryngology at the University of Wisconsin Medical School in Madison. "Don't try to talk over loud noises. And don't try to project your voice at a pitch that's out of your range."

Quench your thirst. "Drink a lot of fluids," says David Alessi, M.D., assistant clinical professor of otolaryngology at the University of California, Los Angeles, UCLA School of Medicine. "If your throat becomes dry, it will hurt even more." He recommends at least eight glasses of water a day.

Get steamed. You can also keep your throat tissue moist with the help of steam, says Barry C. Baron, M.D., associate clinical

When to See the Doctor

S ore throat pain that lasts more than three days should be brought to your doctor's attention, experts say. You should also see your doctor if your sore throat is accompanied by any of the following symptoms.

• Difficulty breathing, swallowing, or opening your mouth
• A fever above 101°F
• Blood in the saliva or phlegm
• Rash
• A lump in your neck
• Earache
• Joint pain

In addition anyone over age 50 with a history of smoking or excessive alcohol consumption should consult a doctor if pain is persistent and progressive, says Charles N. Ford, M.D., professor and chairman of otolaryngology at the University of Wisconsin Medical School in Madison. Both habits greatly increase a person's risk of throat cancer. Likewise, anytime a child has sore throat pain, he should be examined by a doctor. It could be a sign of strep throat, which can lead to rheumatic fever in children.

professor of otolaryngology at the University of California, San Francisco, School of Medicine. He suggests that you run hot water in your kitchen or bathroom sink, then drape a towel over your head to trap the steam and inhale. "Or you could just turn up the hot water in the shower to create a steam bath," he says.

Add moisture to the air. Dry air can aggravate a sore throat. "Try running a humidifier while you sleep," Dr. Alessi suggests. "And use it any time you can during the day."

Have some tea, honey. Tea with honey is a traditional sore throat remedy. You can boost its therapeutic benefits with this spicy twist offered by Cynthia M. Watson, M.D., a family practitioner in private practice in Santa Monica, California: Stir into your tea 1 table-spoon of honey and the juice of half a lemon, then add ground red pepper to taste. "The pepper probably has a mild anesthetic effect," she says. "It also stimulates the immune system."

Think twice about gargling. "Gargling can actually aggra-vate and prolong a sore throat," says Dr. Ford. "Doing it once or twice with salt water might make you feel better by increasing blood flow to the throat area. But doing it regularly—especially with mouthwash—can be very irritating." If you opt for an occasional saltwater rinse, ex-perts suggest a solution of ¼ teaspoon of salt in ½ cup of water. Just be sure to only rinse with, not swallow, the salt water.

Feast on a frozen treat. At last here is a reason that you should eat dessert. Sucking on an ice pop can take the sting out of sore throat pain. "It's cold, it's a fluid, and it tastes good besides," Dr. Janiger notes.

Line up a lozenge. Not all throat lozenges are created equal, experts say. Dr. Alessi contends that the best ones contain glycerine. "It keeps the throat tissue well-hydrated," he explains. You may find these lozenges at health food stores or specialty drugstores.

Dr. Alessi also recommends avoiding lozenges that contain ei-ther mint or menthol. "Both ingredients tend to be drying and are bad for the larynx," he says.

Pick a pill. Both acetaminophen and ibuprofen are recom-mended by experts for an ordinary sore throat. Whichever pain reliever you choose, "take it around the clock according to the package direc-tions on the first day that your throat hurts—even if it seems to get better," Dr. Alessi suggests. "After that, take the medication as needed."

Swallow, don't suck. If you take an aspirin, don't hold it in your mouth for an extended period of time. "Sucking on it may give you some initial relief," says Dr. Alessi. "But it can also irritate the tissue and can cause an acid burn."

Treat your beak. A stuffed-up nose can force you to breathe through your mouth, which irritates your throat, explains Salah D.

Salman, M.D., director of the Sinus Center at the Massachusetts Eye and Ear Infirmary in Boston. So taking an over-the-counter deconges-tant may help ease your sore throat as well, he says.

Address any allergies. Common allergies can cause post-nasal drip, which irritates the throat. "A throat that's itchy—not just painful—points to an allergic condition," Dr. Baron says. "If you have an allergy, an over-the-counter antihistamine may help relieve your symptoms." Antihistamines can have a drying effect, so be sure to in-crease your fluid intake while you're on the medication, he adds. They can also make you drowsy.

Favor mildly flavored foods. "Avoid eating anything that could irritate your throat even more," says Dr. Baron. "Try to stick with bland foods at mild temperatures."

Don't smoke. "Smoking is an irritant," Dr. Ford says. "And it's even more irritating if the throat tissue is already inflamed."

Splinters

Isn't it amazing how much pain something as tiny as a splinter can cause? That shard of wood (or even glass or metal) slips under your skin so stealthily. Then once it's in place, it raises such a ruckus that it feels like a major wound instead of just a misplaced sliver.

What makes splinters so frustrating is that they're seldom easy to get at. They tend to go just far enough beneath the surface of your skin that you have to do some digging to get them out. If you're not careful or if you're a tad less than dexterous, you can irritate or pierce the surrounding skin. You'll end up hurting even more—and you could possibly develop an infection.

Want Relief? Say "Tweeze"

Removing a splinter is easy, once you know how to do it right. It's also the best way to put an end to your pain. Here is how the experts say you should do it.

Clean up. Before you do any poking around, wash the area where the splinter is embedded, advises Joseph A. Witkowski, M.D., clinical professor of dermatology at the University of Pennsylvania School of Medicine and professor of dermatology at the Pennsylvania College of Podiatric Medicine, both in Philadelphia. This will help prevent infection.

Go numb. Rub the area around the splinter with ice, Dr. Witkowski says. "Ice works as a topical anesthetic. It will help reduce your discomfort."

Be well-equipped. Make sure you have the right instrument for splinter removal. In most cases ordinary household tweezers will

When to See the Doctor

It's rare that a splinter requires medical attention, but there are circumstances in which it may be necessary. "If you can't remove a splinter and it hurts, see your doctor," advises Jerome Z. Litt, M.D., assistant clinical professor of dermatology at Case Western Reserve University School of Medicine in Cleveland. "A splinter under your fingernail, for example, can be very difficult to get out. And it will cause more pain there than anywhere else."

You should also see your doctor if you develop an infection, says Libby Bradshaw, D.O., assistant professor of family medicine and community health at Tufts University School of Medicine in Boston. The site of the splinter may fester and become inflamed because there are bacteria on the embedded object, she explains. "You should have the splinter looked at, especially if there is a lot of redness around it or there are red streaks emanating from it," she advises.

do, Dr. Witkowski says. "The kind used for plucking eyebrows works best. You want one with a flat surface rather than a pointed surface. That way, you'll get a better grip on the splinter."

If your splinter proves stubborn, you may want to try a splinter forceps instead, says Libby Bradshaw, D.O., assistant professor of family medicine and community health at Tufts University School of Medicine in Boston. "The forceps has a very sharp, pointed tip that's wonderful for pulling out splinters," she says. "It's a great addition to a home first-aid kit." If you don't already have a splinter forceps, you can buy one in a surgical supply store.

Kill those germs. Whichever tool you choose to use, make sure it is sterilized. Dr. Witkowski suggests wiping your tweezers or splinter forceps with alcohol.

Or you can hold it in a flame, says Jerome Z. Litt, M.D., assistant clinical professor of dermatology at Case Western Reserve University School of Medicine in Cleveland. "Be sure to let the implement cool to room temperature before you use it," he cautions.

Take the right angle. Once you grab the splinter with the tweezers or forceps, carefully pull it out at the same angle it went in. "This will help you avoid breaking the splinter off," Dr. Witkowski says. "You want to pull it out without leaving any part of it behind."

Go for a soak. If you can't get the splinter out completely or if it's stuck, a good soak may help dislodge it, Dr. Witkowski says. He suggests immersing the affected area in warm, soapy water for 5 to 10 minutes, three or four times a day, until the splinter lets go.

Stomach Pain

We tend to blame our tummies for all of our midsection maladies. Think about it: When was the last time you heard someone complain of an upset colon? Or grumble about a gallbladder ache?

Yet what we usually describe as stomach pain may have absolutely nothing to do with the stomach. The abdominal cavity houses a number of organs—including the liver, appendix, intestines, and pancreas—as well as an array of muscles and ducts. Any one of these parts could be causing problems.

Of course, mistaking the onset of appendicitis for a little tummy trouble could have serious consequences. That's why it's so important to be certain of the source of your distress.

As a rule of thumb, experts say, any stomach pain that lasts for more than 24 hours warrants medical attention. If a visit to your doctor is necessary, you may want to do a little pre-exam homework by asking yourself the following questions.

1. How would you describe your pain? Is it gnawing? Burning? Aching? Cramping?
2. Is it steady or intermittent?
3. What makes it better? What makes it worse?
4. Exactly where is it? Above or below your navel? Toward the right or left side of your body?
5. Is it worse when you jostle your body?
6. Does it disrupt your sleep?
7. Do you have other symptoms such as fever, rectal bleeding, vomiting, constipation, or diarrhea?

This information can help guide your doctor to an accurate diagnosis so that you're sure to get the correct treatment for your condition.

Banish That Bellyache

Fortunately, most stomach pain is minor. Often, you can trace it to something you ate—or something you didn't eat. (Experts say that skipping meals can also bring out the beast in your belly.) Or it could be stress that is causing your discomfort. But no matter what its cause, here are some things that you can do to help silence a kvetching stomach.

Don't feed your pain. Sometimes a temperamental tummy just needs a break from its digestive duties. "If you have a cramping pain, don't test it with food," says Roger Gebhard, M.D., professor of medicine at the University of Minnesota in Minneapolis. "You want to avoid stimulating the gastrointestinal tract."

Nausea is another symptom that is better left unfed—which might be a good thing. "If you're nauseated, you won't want to eat or drink anyway," says Naurang Agrawal, M.D., professor of medicine at the University of Connecticut School of Medicine in Farmington.

Get rid of the grumblies. Of course, if you have hunger pangs, by all means eat, advises Dr. Gebhard. When your stomach is empty, all of that unemployed acid—which is normally digesting food may be playing havoc with your stomach lining. "Eating temporarily neutralizes the acid that's in the stomach at the time," he explains.

Choose your chow carefully. Feeding an upset stomach can be tricky. "If you have indigestion, you want to avoid any foods that could aggravate your symptoms," advises Lawrence S. Friedman, M.D., associate professor of medicine at Harvard Medical School. Fatty foods and spicy foods are common troublemakers, he says, but nothing is universally bad or good. "One man's meat is another man's poison," he observes.

You'll have to do some experimenting: If you notice that you feel even worse after eating a particular food, you'll know to stay away from it until you're better. This process can also help you determine which foods are causing your stomach pain in the first place, Dr. Friedman notes.

When to See the Doctor

Any of the following symptoms should send you to your doctor right away.

- Pain accompanied by a change in bowel habits or sudden weight loss
- Bloody or black, tarry stool
- Bloody vomit
- Pain accompanied by a high fever, especially if the fever persists for more than a day or two
- A yellowish hue to the skin or the whites of the eyes
- Pain when you walk
- Recurrent cramping, especially if the episodes become more frequent or more severe
- Pain that disrupts your sleep

Also, be sure to see your doctor if you have persistent stomach pain. How long you wait before seeking medical attention depends, in part, on your overall physical condition, says Lawrence S. Friedman, M.D., associate professor of medicine at Harvard Medical School. Most experts suggest a window of 24 hours.

Stop milking it. If drinking milk or eating ice cream seems to fuel your digestive distress, you may be lactose intolerant. This means that your body isn't producing enough of the enzyme needed to process lactose, the sugar found in milk and milk products.

Try giving up dairy foods to see if it makes a difference. You'll need to do some detective work, though, if you want to dispel all of the lactose from your diet. "You may not be aware of how often you take in lactose," points out Marvin Schuster, M.D., former director of the division of digestive diseases at Johns Hopkins Bayview Medical Center in Baltimore. "It's common to a lot of different foods." Remember to read labels on packaged foods and look for ingredients such as butter, milk, or whey, he says. It's also a good idea to talk to your doctor.

Don't overdo it. It may seem obvious, but it's worth emphasizing: When you're nursing a stomachache, the last thing that you want to do is overeat—especially rich, heavy foods. "Meals should be as light, simple, and easily digested as possible," says Sidney F. Phillips, M.D., professor of medicine at the Mayo Clinic in Rochester, Minnesota.

Eat more fibrous fare. If you have recurrent stomachaches, increasing your fiber intake may help control your symptoms, says David Peura, M.D., associate professor of medicine at the University of Virginia Health Sciences Center in Charlottesville. "Fiber is like a sponge," he explains. "If stools tend to be on the loose side, fiber sops up the extra water. And when it's taken with water, it adds bulk to stools," which triggers the urge to move your bowels.

Just be sure to increase your fiber intake gradually—especially if you're not accustomed to eating a lot of high-fiber foods. "Overdoing it can actually bring on symptoms," Dr. Gebhard notes. "You're putting a load into the bowel. If there are any narrow spots in the bowel, it might prove counterproductive."

Fill up on fluids. It's important to keep up your fluid intake—especially if you have diarrhea, Dr. Gebhard says. "You want to avoid becoming dehydrated," he explains. "You might try Gatorade or another drink with electrolytes in it." Electrolytes are nutrients that regulate your body's chemical balance.

If you're having difficulty drinking because of excessive vomiting, see your physician, urges Dr. Phillips.

Reach for an old standby. Folks have long relied on antacids to ease their digestive distress. These products work well for short-term aches caused by eating or drinking too much, according to Dr. Agrawal.

Note: Don't use an antacid if you're vomiting a lot, Dr. Phillips cautions.

Try something new. Some experts believe that acid inhibitors (such as Tagamet HB)—which are now available over the counter—may be even more effective than antacids in helping to re-

lieve stomach pain. "Antacids neutralize stomach acid. H_2-blockers actually prevent the stomach from making acid," Dr. Peura notes.

Ease diarrhea. If you have diarrhea in addition to pain, Dr. Phillips recommends taking an over-the-counter anti-diarrheal medication (such as Imodium).

Subdue stress. "Anxiety is often a component of digestive disorders," says Mark Goulston, M.D., assistant clinical professor of psychiatry at the University of California, Los Angeles, UCLA School of Medicine and author of *Get Out of Your Own Way*. It can grow from anticipation of a stressful event such as an IRS audit or an important presentation at work—or any situation that makes you feel powerless and out of control.

One way to dodge this emotional distress—and the tummy trouble that accompanies it—is to do some mental rehearsal for the event. "The more prepared you are, the more in control you'll feel, and the less anxiety and pain you'll experience," says Dr. Goulston. He suggests imagining the worst-case scenario. "Be very specific and think of all of the bad things that can happen," he says. "Then decide how you'll handle them if they occur." If you can, enlist the advice of others who have been in similar situations.

Admit your anger. Stomachaches can also result from unexpressed anger, says Dr. Goulston. "Cramping pain is often described as a fist in the stomach," he notes. "Psychologically, there's probably someone that you're mad at or irritated with—someone you wish you could hit." If you feel a fist in your stomach, he says, ask yourself "Whom would I like to punch and why?" It may be another person, or it may be yourself.

Rein in rage. Acknowledging your anger can relieve digestive distress. Constantly losing your temper can make it worse. You can nip emotional outbursts in the bud by learning how to convert anger into conviction, Dr. Goulston says. "Analyze what is making you mad and what moral or ethical principle is being violated," he suggests. "If you stand up for the principle instead of just personal hurt, you'll be able to take more constructive action. And when you start

doing something about the situation, the psychosomatic symptoms—including stomach pain—often go away."

Keep a diary. To help you identify what precipitates your stomachaches, you may want to try writing down everything you eat as well as all of the stress-producing situations you face, advises Dr. Schuster. "When you get pain, review what you have eaten and what has been going on in your life during the previous 12 hours," he says. But don't assume from one isolated incident that a particular food or stressor is responsible for your discomfort. "Something has to happen two or three times so there is consistency," he says. If you notice such a pattern, then avoid the offender to see if your symptoms subside.

Stubbed Toe

This little piggy went to market. This little piggy stayed home. This little piggy smashed into the bedpost—and you sat up the rest of the night, crying and cursing the throbbing digit.

For all the pain they cause stubbed toes have a hard time being taken seriously. Part of the problem is that they are usually self-inflicted, most likely when you're trying to navigate a darkened room in the middle of the night. The fact that "it's just your toe" doesn't help a whole lot either.

Well, maybe this little statistic will finally earn stubbed toes some respect: Researchers have determined that a toe is moving at a speed of 40 to 50 miles per hour when it collides with, say, a table leg. Imagine a car colliding with your foot and you get the idea.

This explains why stubbing your toe can do so much damage. "You can tear soft tissue or a tendon around a toe joint or the metatarsal joint, which is where the toe attaches to the foot," says Phyllis Ragley, D.P.M., a podiatrist in Lawrence, Kansas, and president of the American Academy of Podiatric Sportsmedicine. "You can even break a bone."

So while you may joke about a stubbed toe, it's really nothing to snub. "People blow it off," says Rock Positano, D.P.M., co-director of the Foot and Ankle Orthopedic Institute at the Hospital for Special Surgery in New York City. "Then four or five years later, the toe is killing them. It turns out there's a fracture line and arthritis."

Take Care of That Toe

To be on the safe side, experts say, you should have your doctor examine your stubbed toe. That way you can be sure you haven't done

When to See the Doctor

You should have a stubbed toe looked at by your doctor as soon as possible, experts say. You want to make sure you haven't broken a bone. If a break goes undetected, it can eventually lead to degenerative arthritis and other complications, according to Rock Positano, D.P.M., co-director of the Foot and Ankle Orthopedic Institute at the Hospital for Special Surgery in New York City.

Any of the following symptoms warrants immediate medical attention, adds David C. Novicki, D.P.M., president of the American College of Foot and Ankle Surgeons.

- Marked, persistent swelling, with discoloration that extends up toward the ankle
- Difficulty bearing weight on the toe
- Abnormal positioning of the toe

any serious damage. Until you can get to your doctor—or once he has given you the all clear—these tips can tame your throbbing toe.

Just chill. "Apply ice to your toe right away," says Glenn Gastwirth, D.P.M., deputy executive director of the American Podiatric Medical Association. "The sooner you do so, the sooner you'll reduce the swelling. That's important because swelling puts pressure on the tissues, which in turn puts pressure on the nerves within the tissues. And that contributes a great deal to the pain."

Dr. Ragley suggests massaging the toe with an ice cube for 10 to 15 minutes every hour or two. "But don't do this if you have diabetes or a circulatory problem," she cautions. "The ice can limit circulation in your toe."

Put a hold on heat. Don't use any type of heat treatment on a stubbed toe, advises David C. Novicki, D.P.M., president of the American College of Foot and Ankle Surgeons. "Anything hot will immediately dilate torn blood vessels," he says. "That will lead to the buildup of fluid in the toe."

Attend to a broken nail. The impact between toe and immovable object can cause the nail to tear or break off. "If the nail is still partially attached, cover it with an adhesive bandage to give it a chance to reseat itself," says Dr. Ragley. "If it doesn't reattach or fall off within a few days, clip off the wobbly end."

Keep it up. "Stay off your feet as much as you can—especially for the first 24 to 36 hours after the injury," Dr. Ragley says. "And keep your toe elevated, even if you just have your foot resting on a box 6 inches off the floor. What you don't want is for your foot to be hanging down, with blood running into it. That will increase swelling."

Leave your toe unwrapped. Don't bandage a stubbed toe yourself, Dr. Ragley advises. "You may not wrap it correctly—and if it's fractured, you may do more harm than good," she says. Leave this step to the professionals.

Loosen your bedding. Before you hit the sack, untuck your sheets and blankets so that they put less pressure on your toe, Dr. Gastwirth says. "Downward pressure can bend your toe and add to the soreness," he explains.

Open wide. Make sure your shoe provides ample space for your injured toe, Dr. Ragley says. Choose an open-toed slipper or a sandal over a closed shoe. This will help protect your toe from additional pressure, she explains.

Choose stiff shoes. "Wear a shoe that has a less flexible sole," Dr. Gastwirth says. "It will act much like a splint or a cast, preventing your toe from bending. Your toe will heal much faster if it doesn't bend so much."

Tread carefully. Until you have your toe examined, try not to bend it or put pressure on it when you walk, Dr. Gastwirth says. "You could have a hairline fracture, and pressure would enlarge the crack and possibly displace the bone," he explains. "Shift your weight to your heel as much as possible."

But don't overdo it, he cautions. Overcompensating could cause problems elsewhere in the foot or in the knee or hip.

Sunburn

The sun warms you, relaxes you, brightens your mood. But get too much, and you could end up with an agonizing burn. You can blame a too-tanned hide on Old Sol's ultraviolet (UV) rays. They destroy cells in the outer layer of your skin and damage tiny blood vessels just below the surface. This produces the redness, swelling, and pain that you normally think of when you hear the word *sunburn.*

While the inflammation subsides with time, a sunburn does have long-term effects. "A burn is an injury to your skin, and the damage from it is cumulative," notes Bryan C. Schultz, M.D., clinical associate professor at Loyola University of Chicago Stritch School of Medicine. Repeated overexposure to the sun erodes elastic fibers in your skin, causing wrinkles. Even more serious, it could set the stage for skin cancer.

Overdone by the Sun

Some people are more prone to sunburn than others: Those with fair skin have the highest risk, while African-Americans have the lowest. But no one is completely immune to the sun's savagery.

When fun in the sun leaves your skin scorched, the following strategies can help ease your pain—and keep you from getting burned again.

Put it in neutral. A cold compress helps neutralize a sunburn, according to Steven Earl Prawer, M.D., clinical associate professor of dermatology at the University of Minnesota Medical School in Minneapolis. To make the compress, dip a washcloth or towel in cool tap water, wring it out, and lay it on your skin. "As the water

When to See the Doctor

You can usually treat a mild sunburn—which is mainly redness of the skin—on your own, says Steven Earl Prawer, M.D., clinical associate professor of dermatology at the University of Minnesota Medical School in Minneapolis. "But if the redness covers a large part of your body such as your back, chest, and abdomen, you should see your doctor," he advises.

You should also consult your doctor if your skin blisters or if you experience light-headedness or fainting, Dr. Prawer says. The latter two symptoms may mean that you're dehydrated.

evaporates, it has a cooling effect, which helps control the burning and pain," he explains. He recommends ½-hour applications two or three times a day.

Coat it with cream. One percent hydrocortisone cream (available over the counter) helps relieve sunburn pain, Dr. Prawer says. "Use it directly on the affected area three or four times a day," he advises. "And don't wash it off—just leave it on and keep reapplying it." For added benefit he suggests first applying the cream and then placing a cool compress over the top.

Pop a pain reliever. "Both ibuprofen and aspirin can ease the pain and inflammation of a mild sunburn," according to Dr. Schultz. A more severe burn may require a prescription-strength anti-inflammatory or corticosteroid. "These can have gastrointestinal side effects, though," he says. "Ask your doctor about them."

Hold 'em high. A burn on your lower legs and ankles can cause a lot of swelling, Dr. Schultz says. To prevent that, he suggests keeping your feet elevated as much as possible. Ideally, they should be higher than the level of your heart.

Bathe with care. To cleanse sunburned skin, use relatively cool water and a mild hypoallergenic soap such as Cetaphil or

Oilatum, Dr. Prawer suggests. "Don't scrub your skin or use a wash-cloth," he says. "And if you take a shower, aim the spray away from the affected area."

Read the label. Some ointments intended for sunburn relief contain allergy-causing ingredients, Dr. Schultz says. "Skin that's in-flamed is more susceptible to an allergic reaction," he explains. "It af-fects only a small number of people—but when you have a sunburn, you don't want to experience an allergic reaction besides." If you're allergy-prone, you may want to ask your doctor or pharmacist to rec-ommend a product.

Dress light. You don't want to wear anything that can irritate sunburned skin. "Choose loose clothing made from soft cotton fabric," Dr. Schultz advises. Wool and synthetic fabrics should be avoided until the burn heals.

Safeguard your skin. To prevent another burn, always wear sunscreen when you head outdoors, Dr. Schultz says. He recommends a product with a sun protection factor (SPF) of at least 15. "Apply it ½ hour to 1 hour before you go out so it can soak in," he says. "And take it with you so you can reapply it."

This goes for waterproof sunscreen, too. "If you perspire or go in for swim, some of the sunscreen's effectiveness will be lost," Dr. Schultz says. "No product is absolutely waterproof."

Wear added protection. The proper attire can protect your skin from the sun's UV rays. Tight-knit fabrics work especially well, Dr. Prawer says. But be sure to keep your clothing dry. "If it's wet, about 50 percent of the UV rays will filter through," he notes.

Don't forget your head. Wear a hat to keep the sun off your head and face. "Choose one with a visor or a brim that goes all the way around," Dr. Prawer suggests.

Follow your shadow. The sun's UV rays are at their most in-tense—and therefore do the most damage—between the hours of 10:00 A.M. and 3:00 P.M. Experts advise that you limit your sun expo-sure during this time.

Don't Get Burned

Here are some statistics on Old Sol that can help you save your skin from his damaging ultraviolet (UV) rays.

- Sunlight is at its most intense between the hours of 10:00 A.M. and 3:00 P.M.
- The intensity increases as you head south toward the equator.
- Intensity also increases by about 4 percent for every 1,000 feet in altitude. So if you're skiing at 5,000 feet, for example, the sun's rays are 20 percent stronger.
- Speaking of skiing . . . snow reflects about 85 percent of the sun's UV rays. Sand and concrete reflect about 50 percent.
- A thin cloud cover limits UV radiation by only 20 to 40 percent. In other words you can still get a sunburn when it's cloudy.

So what if you're not wearing a watch? Then heed the short-shadow rule instead. "You can judge the sun's intensity by the length of your shadow," Dr. Schultz explains. "When your shadow is shorter than you, the sun is at its most intense."

Take a raincheck on tanning. Forget the notion that a tan will protect your skin from further damage. "Tanning *is* damage," Dr. Schultz points out. "And it offers skin only the smallest degree of protection."

Temporomandibular Disorder (TMD)

Whoever dubbed it "temporomandibular disorder" must have had a slightly warped sense of humor. After all, you would think that a condition that has jaw pain as one of its symptoms would have a name that's less of a mouthful. Just saying the phrase can sure give your facial muscles a workout—not exactly what you have in mind when you can barely open and close your mouth in the first place.

Mercifully, the condition also goes by its abbreviation: TMD. The TM part refers to the temporomandibular joint, a hingelike structure that enables your jaw to move up and down and from side to side. You can feel the joint when you place a finger just in front of each ear and open and close your mouth.

Every time you chew, swallow, speak, yawn, clench your jaw, or grind your teeth, your temporomandibular joint is called into service. It's easy to see why the joint is so susceptible to wear and tear and injury.

If you have difficulty moving your jaw, feel pain when chewing, or notice grating or clicking sounds in the area of your temporomandibular joint, you may indeed have TMD. You may also experience TMD-related symptoms in your eyes, ears, face, head, neck, and shoulders.

Tempering TMD

Treatment for TMD runs the gamut from simple self-care techniques to sophisticated surgical procedures. Most experts recommend pursuing the more conservative pain-relief options first. "Rushing into

255

an aggressive or irreversible treatment such as surgery or tooth adjustment is usually not necessary and can be counterproductive," says Steven Syrop, D.D.S., director of the TMD–facial pain program at Columbia University School of Dental and Oral Surgery in New York City.

The following remedies can help ease your TMD pain.

Bring on the big chill. Experts recommend cold applications to the affected area at the onset of pain. A bag of frozen peas works exceptionally well for this purpose, says Ira Klemons, D.D.S., Ph.D., director of the Center for Head and Facial Pain in South Amboy, New Jersey. "It conforms to the contours of your face, so it's not as uncomfortable as regular ice," he explains. "Wrap the bag in a towel and leave it in place for 10 minutes, then wait an hour before reapplying."

Heat things up. After two to three days of cold applications, you can begin treating your TMD with heat, Dr. Klemons says. Heat supports the healing process by relaxing the muscles and enhancing circulation. "Use a heating pad or a hot-water bottle with a moist washcloth underneath it," he advises. He recommends a 10-minute application once every hour.

You should never apply heat immediately at the onset of pain, Dr. Klemons adds. "It can increase blood flow to the affected area and make matters worse."

Be a softy. While you're nursing an aching jaw, you will want to steer clear of crunchy, chewy foods, experts say. That means giving up nuts, tough meats, hard breads—any foods that overwork your jaw and its adjacent muscles.

But that doesn't give you permission to forgo your good eating habits. "Don't limit yourself to unhealthy soft foods," Dr. Klemons says. "There are good foods that are soft, such as yogurt, cottage cheese, and soup. And make sure that you're getting enough protein and complex carbohydrates."

Downsize your bites. "Cut your food into small pieces," advises Joan Schmidt, director of Westwood Physical Therapy in Los Angeles. "And avoid items that require you to open your mouth wide or bite with your front teeth, such as apples and club sandwiches."

> ## Loosening a Locked Jaw
>
> For some unlucky folks temporomandibular disorder has a nasty habit of making the jaw lock in place. "It's usually caused by a muscle going into spasm," explains Ira Klemons, D.D.S., Ph.D., director of the Center for Head and Facial Pain in South Amboy, New Jersey. Here's what he suggests you do if this should happen to you: Go to a quiet room, sit down, and close your eyes. Relax and count to 60 in your head. "This prevents a panic reaction—which would make the problem worse—and allows your jaw to slip back into its normal position," he says.

Give both sides equal time. It's unwise to speak from both sides of your mouth, but it's a good idea to chew that way, experts say. "Chew symmetrically on each side," says Schmidt. "And use your back teeth, not your front ones."

Don't gum up the works. This is definitely not the time to find out whether you can still fit an entire pack of bubblegum in your mouth at once, as you could in high school. "Avoid chewing gum unless your doctor or physical therapist tells you otherwise," says Schmidt.

Keep nervous nibbling in check. "Habits like gnawing on pencils or the earpieces of your eyeglasses overuse the temporomandibular joint," says Dr. Syrop. "It's kind of like having a sprained ankle and running on it all day."

Drink decaf. "Avoid caffeine, whether in coffee, tea, or cola," Schmidt advises. "It can make the muscles in the area of your jaw even more tense."

Don't get puffed up. Puffing on a cigarette, cigar, or pipe forces you to protrude your lower jaw, Schmidt observes. And that can make TMD pain even worse.

What's more, "smokers are more sensitive to pain than nonsmokers," Dr. Klemons says. "They heal more slowly, too."

Mind your makeup routine. "Many women apply lipstick to the bottom lip, then get it on the upper lip by rolling their lips together," Schmidt says. "When they do that, they protrude the lower jaw"—not a wise move when you have TMD. She recommends using a lipstick brush instead.

Unhand your jaw. Remember how Jack Benny would cup his jaw in his hand? That's a no-no for anyone with TMD. "You're applying more pressure to the temporomandibular joint," Schmidt explains. "It's also a very bad position for the neck—and people with TMD often have neck problems as well."

Don't yield to yawning. When you have TMD, something as ordinary as a yawn can cause considerable discomfort. It can make your jaw lock, too, Schmidt says. "When you feel a yawn coming on, place your tongue on the roof of your mouth and slowly bend your head forward," she suggests. "This puts less mechanical tension on the joint."

Hold the phone. "Don't cradle the receiver of your phone against your shoulder," says Dr. Klemons. "It puts tremendous strain on the muscles of your head, face, and neck."

Quit the daily (and nightly) grind. Tooth grinding can cause TMD and aggravate the resulting ache. You should make a conscious effort to stop this pain-producing habit, Dr. Syrop says. "Remember the phrase 'Lips together, teeth apart,' " he suggests. "Put little self-stick notes around your home and office to remind yourself."

If you grind your teeth while you sleep, Dr. Klemons recommends doing this exercise before you go to bed: Bite as hard as you can for 6 seconds, then completely relax for 6 seconds. Then do it again—bite, relax, bite, relax, for a total of three times each. "Many people find that within a few days they stop clenching," he says.

Try a mouthpiece. Wearing a mouthpiece can provide relief from TMD by preventing you from grinding your teeth, Dr. Klemons says. You can purchase one in a sporting goods store. He recommends

---

When to See the Doctor

If you have pain in your temporomandibular joint because of an accidental injury, don't wait to seek medical attention, advises Ira Klemons, D.D.S., Ph.D., director of the Center for Head and Facial Pain in South Amboy, New Jersey. You should also see a doctor if you experience any of the following symptoms.
- Pain in your temples, jaw, or temporomandibular joint
- Difficulty opening your mouth more than 1½ inches
- Clicking or grating sounds when you open your mouth

Be sure to choose a physician who is qualified to treat temporomandibular disorder (TMD), Dr. Klemons says. Contact you local hospital for a referral to a qualified professional in your area. "Members of the association who are diplomates or fellows have passed rigorous exams and have extensive experience with TMD," he says.

wearing it while you sleep and any other time that's convenient for you. "But if you're not dramatically better in two to four weeks, stop wearing it and see a doctor," he says.

Fortify with supplements. "A deficiency in thiamin, vitamin B_6, or vitamin B_{12} can increase your susceptibility to muscle pain," Schmidt says. She recommends getting at least 50 milligrams of each of these nutrients per day, along with regular doses of vitamin C. "Five hundred milligrams with each meal helps decrease muscle stiffness," she observes.

Note: Taking more than 1,200 milligrams of vitamin C a day may cause diarrhea in some people.

Ease the pain with aspirin. Experts recommend aspirin or another nonsteroidal anti-inflammatory drug (NSAID) to help reduce inflammation in the temporomandibular joint. But if you find it necessary to continue the medication for an extended period of time, you should see your doctor, Dr. Klemons says.

Work your muscles. Dr. Syrop recommends this TMD-taming routine: Begin by gently massaging the muscles in the affected area for 5 seconds. Then stretch the muscles by opening your mouth, but not to the point of pain. Hold for 5 seconds. Repeat the cycle of massaging for 5 seconds and stretching for 5 seconds five times. Do this five times a day, Dr. Syrop says—"but not if it hurts."

Make your point. Applying pressure to a point between your thumb and index finger can ease TMD pain, Dr. Klemons says. To find the point, put your thumb and index finger together. You'll notice the formation of a crease and, above it, a small bump. Put the thumb of your opposite hand on the bump, then separate your thumb and index finger. Press on that point firmly for about a minute, then switch to your other hand. You should feel some relief, he says. "If the pain comes back, do it again."

Teach yourself to relax. Stress contributes to TMD pain, Dr. Klemons says. Practicing a relaxation technique can prevent you from tensing your jaw in stressful situations. Studies have shown meditation to be especially effective for this purpose, he notes. "To the extent that stress aggravates TMD, meditation would have the opposite effect."

Tennis Elbow

You don't have to play tennis to get tennis elbow. In fact, about 95 percent of folks with this condition never set foot on a court. Instead, they garden, they type, they turn wrenches, they carry briefcases—activities that require them to repeatedly rotate the elbow or flex the wrist, usually while gripping a heavy object.

Like a good backhand, tennis elbow—or lateral epicondylitis, in medical lingo—takes time to develop. The first sign is usually soreness or a dull ache on the outside of the elbow joint that gets worse when you grasp something. Eventually, the pain may radiate down the top of your forearm, sometimes all the way to your wrist.

Take care of tennis elbow promptly, experts advise. Left untreated, it can transform a routine task such as turning a key or picking up a book into an excruciating experience.

Relief, Anyone?

The best thing you can do for an aching elbow is to stop the activity that's aggravating it, says Phillip A. Bauman, M.D., clinical instructor in orthopedic surgery at the Columbia University College of Physicians and Surgeons and associate attending physician of orthopedic surgery at St. Luke's–Roosevelt Hospital Center, both in New York City. But rest isn't the only answer. The following tips can also help you ace elbow pain.

Say "ahhh" with ice. Freeze some water in a paper cup, then peel back the top of the cup and rub the ice on your elbow in a circular motion for 5 to 7 minutes, suggests William S. Case, president of Case Physical Therapy in Houston. Repeat this treatment at least two times a day for the first five days that you have pain, he says.

Don't Blame Your Game

Just because your elbow hurts that doesn't mean you have tennis elbow. The joint is susceptible to an array of other problems, too.

Among the most common is cubital tunnel syndrome, says Phillip A. Bauman, M.D., clinical instructor in orthopedic surgery at the Columbia University College of Physicians and Surgeons and associate attending physician of orthopedic surgery at St. Luke's/Roosevelt Hospital Center, both in New York City. With this condition, the ulnar nerve—the nerve that sends out shock waves of pain when you knock your funny bone on a hard surface—gets trapped in a groove on the inside of the elbow. It may produce a burning or pins-and-needles sensation or pain that shoots down to your fourth and fifth fingers, he says.

Then there's medial epicondylitis, which is much like tennis elbow (or lateral epicondylitis). The difference is that it affects the inside of your arm rather than the outside.

Both of these conditions will respond to the same remedies as tennis elbow. That translates to lots of rest and tender loving care.

Help heal with heat. After five days of applying ice to your elbow, you can switch to warm compresses or soaks, Case says. He suggests 15-minute treatment sessions, two or three times a day.

Think ginger. To spice up your heat treatment, try a ginger compress, says Arthur H. Brownstein, M.D., a physician in Princeville, Hawaii, and clinical instructor of medicine at the University of Hawaii School of Medicine in Manoa. His instructions: Boil some freshly grated gingerroot, then allow it to cool to a tolerable temperature. You want it to be as hot as you can comfortably stand. Then soak a washcloth in the brew and place it over your elbow. The ginger helps draw out toxins and speeds the healing process, he explains.

Try homeopathy. The homeopathic remedy Ruta graveolens can help soothe a sore elbow, says Cynthia M. Watson, M.D., a family practitioner in private practice in Santa Monica, California. She recommends taking a 6X dose every hour while your pain is severe, then three or four times a day as your condition improves. (The notation 6X refers to the remedy's potency, which is indicated on the label.) You will find Ruta graveolens in health food stores and wherever homeopathic remedies are sold.

Stick with an old standby. A nonsteroidal anti-inflammatory drug (NSAID) such as aspirin or ibuprofen can relieve pain and swelling, Dr. Bauman says. But you should stop taking the medication once you resume a normal level of activity. "You want to be aware of any pain that occurs so you know when you're straining the area," he explains.

Use soothing strokes. Relaxing the surrounding muscles can take some of the pressure off an aching elbow, Dr. Brownstein says. "Gently massage the full length of your forearm muscle from your elbow to above your wrist—not just where you feel pain."

Brace yourself. Try an elbow support, Dr. Bauman suggests. "It prevents you from contracting the extensor muscle when you move your hand," he explains. (The extensor muscle pulls on the lateral

---

When to See the Doctor

If your elbow pain is extreme or persists for more than a month, you should consult your doctor, advises Phillip A. Bauman, M.D., clinical instructor in orthopedic surgery at the Columbia University College of Physicians and Surgeons and associate attending physician of orthopedic surgery at St. Luke's/Roosevelt Hospital Center, both in New York City. Also see your doctor if your elbow is red and swollen and you have chills and fever. These symptoms may indicate an infection or a tumor, he says.

epicondyle, a bony protuberance on the forearm that is involved in tennis elbow.) "It also reminds you to give the injured area a rest." You can buy one of these devices in a drugstore or a medical supply store.

Make some muscle. Once your elbow is on the mend, gentle strengthening and stretching exercises can help rehabilitate the joint and protect it from reinjury, experts say. They suggest that you give these moves a try—but only after any pain and inflammation subsides.

- While holding a 2-pound dumbbell (a 2-pound can of soup or vegetables works just as well), rest your forearm on a tabletop, with your wrist extending over the edge and your palm facing down. Slowly raise and lower the dumbbell, moving your wrist through its full range of motion. Repeat 15 to 20 times, then change hands. Do the exercise three times a day. If you experience any pain, try switching to a lighter weight.
- Hold your arm straight out in front of you, with your palm facing down. Make a fist and bend your wrist upward. Try to push the fist down with your other hand. Hold for 10 seconds, then relax. Repeat five times. Perform this exercise two or three times a day, gradually working up to 20 repetitions.

  Note: You need only to work the hand on the arm that has tennis elbow, but you may wish to perform the exercise on both hands.

Pick up where you left off. You can ease back into your normal routine when your elbow no longer bothers you. "As a general rule, there should be no pain associated with day-to-day tasks before you move on to something more demanding," Dr. Bauman says. "Give yourself time to see how your elbow reacts. Don't overdo it just because you don't feel pain right away."

Consult a pro. If you developed tennis elbow because of a particular sport or activity, you may want to have a professional check out your form and technique, says Stella Shigenaka, a physical therapist at the Institute of Progressive Physical Therapy in Los Angeles. A fitness trainer or coach can troubleshoot problems and evaluate your equipment. If you play tennis, for example, a too-heavy racquet or too-thick grip can contribute to tennis elbow.

Testicular Pain

Want to make a grown man cry? All it takes is a poorly aimed softball or a close encounter with a foot. In fact, any kind of blow to the groin can bring even the toughest of tough guys to his knees. The pain is indescribable. Fortunately, it is also short-lived: It usually goes away in just a couple of minutes.

But sometimes the testicles hurt without any apparent provocation. Perhaps the most serious cause of testicular pain is torsion, in which the cord that supplies blood to the testicle becomes twisted. Torsion hurts so badly, experts say, that anyone who has it will head straight for an emergency room. And that's precisely what you should do.

Less serious but more common than torsion is epididymitis, in which the epididymis—a stringlike tube that lies behind the testicle—becomes inflamed. When you have this condition, the testicle may appear swollen and feel tender.

Sometimes testicular pain is referred, meaning the problem lies elsewhere in your body. For example, a kidney stone or a pinched nerve in your lower back may cause your testicles to hurt, explains Dudley Danoff, M.D., senior attending urologist at Cedars–Sinai Medical Center in Los Angeles and author of *Superpotency.*

Try a Little Tenderness

Since testicular pain could signal a serious problem—especially if the pain persists or becomes more intense over time—you should see your doctor as soon as possible for a diagnosis. In the meantime, follow this expert advice for fast, temporary relief.

For an injury, choose ice. If your testicles take a serious blow, apply ice immediately, Dr. Danoff says. "Put some cubes in

When to See the Doctor

If you experience sudden, excruciating pain in a testicle, get to an emergency room as quickly as possible, says Dudley Danoff, M.D., senior attending urologist at Cedars–Sinai Medical Center in Los Angeles and author of *Superpotency.* You may have a torsion. "Torsion requires immediate medical attention because it deprives the testicle of blood," he explains. And without blood the testicle can deteriorate and die within a matter of hours.

What about testicular cancer? It seldom produces pain, says Stephen Jacobs, M.D., professor of urology at the University of Maryland School of Medicine in Baltimore. But if you notice a lump in a testicle, you should bring it to your doctor's attention.

plastic wrap or a sandwich bag and close it up with a rubber band," he suggests. "Then wrap the pack in a towel or a washcloth." Apply the ice in cycles of 15 minutes on and 10 minutes off. "If the pain doesn't go away in a couple of hours or if it intensifies, get to your doctor without delay," he says. "You may have internal bleeding."

Rest up. Don't do anything too vigorous or jarring, says John J. Mulcahy, M.D., Ph.D., professor of urology at the Indiana University Medical Center in Indianapolis. You want to prevent the scrotum (the "bag" that holds the testicles) from hitting against your thighs when you move around.

Keep them in suspension. A device called a scrotal suspensory can immobilize the testicles when you are on the go, Dr. Mulcahy says. "It's similar to an athletic supporter, but not as tight," he explains. "An athletic supporter creates pressure that will make your pain even worse." You can purchase a scrotal suspensory in a drugstore or medical supply store.

Add some lift. "You can relieve your pain somewhat by elevating your scrotum," says Stephen Jacobs, M.D., professor of urology at the University of Maryland School of Medicine in Baltimore. He suggests using a towel to prop up the testicles while you're sitting down.

Avoid aspirin. "Aspirin is a very potent blood thinner," Dr. Danoff says. "It would cause problems if you would need to have some sort of surgery done." If you want to take a pain reliever, choose ibuprofen instead, he advises.

Be open to antibiotics. If you do have an infection such as epididymitis, you'll need to take antibiotics to clear it up, according to Dr. Mulcahy. Tetracycline is the usual prescription, he says.

Consider acupuncture. The thought of needles in the groin probably isn't very appealing. But acupuncture has proven to be very successful in treating testicular pain, practitioners say. "From the point of view of Chinese medicine, acupuncture reduces the stagnation that is causing your pain," explains Pamela Miller, a licensed acupuncturist at Balfour Chiropractic in Northridge, California. To locate a qualified acupuncturist in your area, contact the physician referral service of your local hospital.

Tongue Pain

B iting your tongue can be good advice at times—like when your mother-in-law asks you what you think of her new hairdo. But when you take this advice too literally, your attempt at tact may well be rewarded with unspeakable agony.

You probably don't think about your tongue a whole lot until you clamp down on it with your bicuspids. Then you are quickly reminded of what a tender and sensitive organ it is. While bites and other minor injuries are probably the most common cause of tongue pain, they are by no means the only cause.

"Your tongue can hurt in the absence of injury," says Kenneth M. Hargreaves, D.D.S., Ph.D., associate professor in the divisions of endodontics and pharmacology at the University of Minnesota Medical School in Minneapolis. "The lymph nodes under the tongue can become swollen as the result of an infection or even some forms of cancer. The ducts in the salivary glands under the tongue can get blocked." Tongue pain can also be a symptom of allergies or iron deficiency or a side effect of certain medications.

Speak the Language of Relief

Because tongue pain can signal a serious health problem, don't hesitate to see your dentist for a professional diagnosis. But for a more run-of-the-mill sore, burn, or abrasion, the following tips can bring you relief.

Bide your time. Your mouth can heal quite quickly on its own because it has such a quick turnover of cells. For this reason Dr. Hargreaves says, "doing nothing will usually work just fine. Hang in there a few days."

Experts say that you should notice improvement in 7 to 10 days. If you don't, see your dentist.

Choose foods wisely. You can easily aggravate a mouth sore by eating the wrong foods. Most experts recommend avoiding anything salty, spicy, or acidic—and that includes orange juice and tomato juice. You can reduce the acidity of these beverages by diluting them with water, says Lawrence Wolinsky, D.M.D., Ph.D., professor of oral biology at the University of California, Los Angeles, School of Dentistry. That way they won't burn when you swallow them.

Bag the butts. Cigarette smoke is an irritant that can make your tongue pain even worse, says Howard S. Glazer, D.D.S., a dentist in Fort Lee, New Jersey, and past president of the Academy of General Dentistry. You would be much better off if you quit huffing and puffing.

Maintain your routine. While the thought of wielding a toothbrush near your throbbing tongue may make you bristle, it is

Pain That's Aflame

You might have expected a burning sensation had you sipped from a cup of too-hot coffee or chowed down on super-spicy buffalo wings. But you have done neither, and your tongue still feels as though it's on fire.

You could have a condition known as burning tongue syndrome. "It feels as if you're holding a match to your tongue," says Ira Klemons, D.D.S., Ph.D., director of the Center for Head and Facial Pain in South Amboy, New Jersey. "It's a horrible, constant pain."

While burning tongue syndrome has been linked to everything from deficiencies of iron and niacin to menopause, Dr. Klemons has found that it usually accompanies head or facial pain. "At least 70 percent of patients have other symptoms in and about the head and face," he says. And when those symptoms are relieved, the tongue pain tends to go away, too.

Here are a few other culprits that you should be aware of. *Note:* If you suspect that you have burning tongue syndrome, you should see your dentist for proper diagnosis and treatment.

Medications. Antihistamines, antidepressants, tranquilizers, and drugs for high blood pressure and heart problems can all contribute to burning tongue syndrome. "Tell your dentist what kind

more important now than ever. Brushing regularly—the usual recommendation is three to five times a day—will keep your mouth free of food debris.

Rinse and spit. Gargling with warm salt water each time you brush your teeth can provide temporary relief, experts say. If you have high blood pressure or heart disease, be aware that many commercial mouth rinses contain a lot of sodium. To limit the amount you absorb, Dr. Wolinsky says, don't swallow the rinse—just swish it around in your mouth, then spit it out.

of medication you're taking," says Thomas F. Razmus, D.D.S., associate professor in the department of diagnostic services at the West Virginia University School of Dentistry in Morgantown. "You may have to live with burning tongue syndrome because you need the medication, but at least you'll know the source of the problem."

Mouth-care products. A burning tongue can signal an adverse reaction to toothpaste or mouthwash. "A fair number of people have trouble with tartar-control toothpaste," Dr. Razmus notes. "They develop a slimy coating and a burning sensation on their tongues." You might consider changing types or brands of toothpaste or cutting back on mouthwash, using it every other day instead of once a day or more.

Yeast infections. Oral candidiasis—a yeast infection of the mouth—is common in people who have been on long-term antibiotics, says Dr. Razmus. "When you wipe out the 'normal' bacteria in the mouth, the yeast take over, and that can cause a burning tongue," he explains. Talk to your doctor or dentist about weaning yourself from the antibiotic or switching to another kind.

Women who have histories of vaginal yeast infections also seem more prone to oral candidiasis, Dr. Razmus says.

You might also want to talk to your dentist about using a prescription rinse containing lidocaine viscous (such as Xylocaine Viscous). "It's a topical agent for the treatment of sore gums, denture sores, and tongue irritation," Dr. Glazer says. "It can provide short-term pain relief."

Apply an anesthetic. Look for an over-the-counter medication called Orajel, says Thomas F. Razmus, D.D.S., associate professor in the department of diagnostic services at the West Virginia University School of Dentistry in Morgantown. "Orajel is a topical anesthetic, so it will reduce the pain," he says. "And it sticks to wet tissue, so it serves as a protective coating for any lesions in the mouth."

Get checked for deficiencies. "Tongue pain can be a symptom of a nutrient deficiency, usually in the B-complex vitamins," says Dr. Glazer. "It could also indicate anemia." He recommends that you ask your doctor or dentist to run tests to rule out these conditions.

Fix your choppers. A jagged tooth or a poorly fitting denture can make your tongue sore, says Jay W. Friedman, D.D.S., a dental consultant in Los Angeles and author of *Complete Guide to Dental Health*. See your dentist to have the proper repair work done.

Look for suspicious spots. Inspect your tongue in a mirror for any lesion or ulceration. The Academy of General Dentistry recommends that you do this every month or if your tongue is painful. And don't just look at the surface. Check the sides and underneath, too. If you notice something, observe it for a week to 10 days. "If it doesn't go away, have it checked by your dentist—especially if it has no apparent cause," Dr. Friedman says.

A painful sore that can be traced to a specific injury is actually less ominous than a painless one that you don't become aware of until you happen to spot it in the mirror or your dentist notices it during a routine exam. "The more common types of mouth cancer begin without any soreness," Dr. Friedman notes. "That's another reason why it's good to have regular (twice yearly) oral examinations."

Toothache

Maybe that's why it's called a wisdom tooth: Boy, can it smart! Actually, every one of your 32 pearly whites is a tiny time bomb of oral torture, able to produce pain so intolerable that you would do just about anything for relief.

The most common source of dental discomfort is tooth decay. As decay progresses, bacteria invade the pulp the mass of blood vessels and nerves at the center of the tooth—and activate pain receptors there. "It hurts when you bite down or drink something cold," says Kenneth M. Hargreaves, D.D.S., Ph.D., associate professor in the divisions of endodontics and pharmacology at the University of Minnesota Medical School in Minneapolis. "And sometimes it just throbs for no apparent reason."

A cracked tooth also produces pain, but you may feel it only when you bite a certain way. "The pressure of biting opens the crack further," explains Richard Price, D.M.D., clinical instructor at the Henry Goldman School of Dentistry at Boston University.

Then there's dental hypersensitivity, which occurs when tubules that make up a tooth's root are exposed—usually by toothbrush abrasion or erosion. When this happens, Dr. Hargreaves says, sugary sweets, ice-cold beverages, and other fare can stimulate the pain receptors inside the tubules. So every meal becomes an oral obstacle course as you try to maneuver food and drink past the sensitive tooth without triggering an agonizing reaction.

Open Wide and Say "Ahhh"

In general, whenever you have an aching tooth, you should see your dentist as soon as possible so that he can determine what's causing

A Toothache That Isn't

Sometimes you may develop pain in teeth that are perfectly healthy. Doctors call this referred pain, which simply means that the real problem lies in another part of your body. "If you have a dull ache that seems to affect several teeth as opposed to a single tooth, it might be referred from the muscles and joints of the face or head," notes Ira Klemons, D.D.S., Ph.D., director of the Center for Head and Facial Pain in South Amboy, New Jersey.

One common cause of false toothaches is temporomandibular disorder (TMD). Consider whether you're experiencing any of these common TMD symptoms: pain when you compress your jaw, difficulty opening your mouth more than 1½ inches, or clicking or grating sounds when you open and close your mouth. (For a more detailed discussion of this condition, see the chapter on page 255.)

A sinus infection can also mimic a toothache, says Howard S. Glazer, D.D.S., a dentist in Fort Lee, New Jersey, and past president of the Academy of General Dentistry. "It's called maxillary sinusitis," he says. "It's an impingement on the nerve endings of the tooth caused by pressure buildup in the sinus cavity. There's nothing wrong with the tooth itself."

This condition is especially common during winter, when colds are more prevalent, says Richard Price, D.M.D., clinical instructor at the Henry Goldman School of Dentistry at Boston University. But it can occur during the summer, too—especially in people who have allergies.

"The patient can't describe exactly where the pain is," Dr. Price says. "If we can't diagnose the problem, we prescribe a three-day regimen of decongestants. That usually clears it up."

your pain, says Jay W. Friedman, D.D.S., a dental consultant in Los Angeles and author of *Complete Guide to Dental Health*. Once you have scheduled an appointment, try the following tips for temporary relief.

Give up the triggers. The easiest way to alleviate the discomfort of dental hypersensitivity is to stop consuming whatever is causing you problems. "If you experience pain when you eat sweets, for example, then do your best to avoid them," Dr. Hargreaves says.

Ease up a bit. Being physically active is a very good thing. But when you have a toothache, going full steam ahead can actually intensify your pain. "When you move around a lot, your heart pumps harder," says Howard S. Glazer, D.D.S., a dentist in Fort Lee, New Jersey, and past president of the Academy of General Dentistry. "Since your heart and your jaw are so close to each other, an increase in the pumping action of your heart can heighten the pressure in your tooth and possibly aggravate your discomfort."

This doesn't mean that you should lie in bed, he adds. But you might want to limit your activity until you see your dentist.

Be finicky about food. Chewing can stimulate your tooth and make it hurt even more. Dr. Hargreaves suggests that you stick with soft foods and chew on the side of your mouth opposite your sore tooth.

Also, says Dr. Glazer, avoid foods that are spicy or extremely hot or cold.

Wash away pain. Dr. Glazer recommends treating a toothache with frequent saltwater rinses. "Salt is an excellent astringent," he notes. "It draws things out. Use warm—not hot—water, and rinse as often as you can. You can't overdose." Be sure not to swallow the saltwater.

Try oil of cloves. "Oil of cloves contains 80 percent eugenol, which has local anesthetic properties," Dr. Hargreaves says. "It's less expensive than over-the-counter toothache remedies such as Anbesol, which also have local anesthetic properties. It probably won't taste as good, though."

You'll find oil of cloves in health food stores. To use it, Dr. Hargreaves suggests putting a few drops on a cotton ball and then gently biting on the cotton with your sore tooth. "It's most effective in reducing pain if it can get to the affected pain receptors," he explains.

Plug the hole. Oil of cloves also works well as a temporary filling for a tooth that has lost its filling, says Dr. Price. Simply fill the hole with cotton soaked in oil of cloves until you can get to your dentist.

Another good temporary filling is soft orthodontic wax, which you can buy in most drugstores. Gently rinse your tooth and fill the hole with the wax, Dr. Price says. This will protect the tooth from cold water, food, and other elements.

"In a pinch, you can even fill the hole with sugarless chewing gum," Dr. Price adds.

Take a pill. "You can try an over-the-counter oral medication to ease a toothache," says Dr. Hargreaves. "Acetaminophen or a non-steroidal anti-inflammatory drug (NSAID) such as ibuprofen might give you relief."

Get to the point. The time-honored practice of acupressure works quite well in relieving tooth pain, practitioners say. To give it a try, you'll first want to locate the appropriate acupressure point, which lies between the thumb and index finger of either hand. "The point is called *hoku,*" says Irwin Koff, M.D., a general practitioner in Kahuku, Hawaii, who is certified in acupuncture. "It means 'mountain' in Chinese. If you close your thumb and index finger, you'll notice a little rise next to the crease. That's where the point is."

Then, he says, simply press the point on the hand opposite the affected tooth. In other words if the sore tooth is on the left side of your mouth, work the point on your right hand, and vice versa.

Flex your fingers. Manipulating points near the tips of your fingers can also relieve dental pain, says Dean Sluyter, a certified reflexologist in Plainfield, New Jersey. (In reflexology you heal the body by working specific points on the feet and hands.)

According to Sluyter, each finger of each hand equals one or two teeth on your upper or lower jaw—that is, your thumbs correspond to your front teeth, your index fingers to your eyeteeth, and so on. If your toothache is halfway back on the right side of your mouth, you should work the point on the middle finger of your right hand. And if it's a left molar that's hurting, you should work the point on your left pinkie.

When to See the Dentist

If you have a toothache, experts say that you should see your dentist as soon as possible. It's very important to find out exactly what is causing your pain.

What's more, you should keep that appointment even if your toothache goes away on its own, says Jay W. Friedman, D.D.S., a dental consultant in Los Angeles and author of *Complete Guide to Dental Health.* The reason? "Most toothaches result from dental decay," Dr. Friedman explains. "The pain might disappear because the nerve has degenerated. Over time, the tooth might develop an abscess without your knowing about it."

What can you do if a toothache strikes when you're on the road and far from your regular dentist? Call the American Dental Association at 1-800-621-8099, extension 2593, for a referral.

The points themselves are located just below the cuticles of your fingernails. To find the point you want to work, Sluyter says, rest your hand on something stable, like a tabletop. Using the index or middle finger of your other hand, probe just below the cuticle of the finger that corresponds to your sore tooth. Feel for a point that's a little sensitive or tender. Apply steady, firm pressure to it for 30 to 60 seconds. "You usually feel a sudden shift—your finger or your tooth doesn't hurt as much," Sluyter says.

Ulcers

I don't get ulcers. I give them." Sounds like the mean-spirited mantra of some hard-boiled, take-no-prisoners corporate executive, doesn't it? Indeed, ulcers were long considered the domain of hardworking Joes and Janes, who bore the painful sores like badges of honor for toiling 60-plus hours a week in high-stress jobs.

But as researchers have discovered, ulcers are caused not by belligerent bosses or demanding deadlines but by a tough-as-nails bacterium called *Helicobacter pylori.* This spiral-shaped organism invades and then weakens the protective lining of the stomach, impairing the lining's ability to withstand the caustic effects of stomach acid. The acid—which normally aids the digestive process—begins to eat away at the stomach lining itself, leaving behind craterlike lesions.

Bacterial infection is now considered the leading cause of ulcers. Many experts believe that eradicating *H. pylori* in the stomach can not only heal an existing sore but also prevent a future recurrence.

Some people may develop ulcers from the long-term use of nonsteroidal anti-inflammatory drugs (NSAIDs). Like *H. pylori,* these medications make the stomach lining more vulnerable to acid.

What about lifestyle factors such as stress and diet? Once considered the major players in the development of ulcers, they are now relegated to supporting roles. They don't cause ulcers directly, but they can make you more susceptible to the sores and aggravate your symptoms.

Pull the Plug on Pain

An ulcer usually makes its presence known with a gnawing or burning sensation in the abdomen, between the breastbone and the navel. You may notice that the pain goes away when you eat—but

When to See the Doctor

An ulcer produces a gnawing or burning sensation in the upper abdomen, usually on an empty stomach. But having this symptom doesn't necessarily mean that you have an ulcer, says Lawrence S. Friedman, M.D., associate professor of medicine at Harvard Medical School. "It could be a condition that we call non-ulcer dyspepsia," he says. "Essentially, it's indigestion."

If you have persistent symptoms, or if your symptoms don't respond to antacids, you should see your doctor for a diagnostic evaluation. This is especially important if you have any complication such as vomiting, weight loss, or pain when you eat. (Typically, ulcer pain is somewhat relieved by eating.) "And if you're passing blood or vomiting blood, or if your stool is black (the result of digested blood), you should seek medical attention right away," says David Peura, M.D., associate professor of medicine at the University of Virginia Health Sciences Center in Charlottesville.

more than likely it will come back.

If you think you have an ulcer, see your doctor for a proper diagnosis. If he confirms your suspicions, these tips can help minimize your discomfort—and perhaps cure your ulcer for good.

Stay the course. For an ulcer caused by *H. pylori,* your doctor will likely prescribe a course of treatment that heals the sore and kills off the bacteria, says Lawrence S. Friedman, M.D., associate professor of medicine at Harvard Medical School. The most commonly used regimen consists of two weeks of antibiotics, two weeks of bismuth subsalicylate (the active ingredient in Pepto-Bismol), and four to six weeks of an acid blocker. If you follow this regimen, there is an excellent chance that the ulcer won't come back, Dr. Friedman says. "The recurrence rate is less than 10 percent," he notes. "By comparison, if you treat the ulcer but don't eradicate the bacteria, the recurrence rate can be as high as 80 percent."

This is a lot of medication to take, and doctors concede that the antibiotics in particular have potential side effects, including indigestion, nausea, and diarrhea. "These are not insignificant," says Dr. Friedman. "But the temporary discomfort is worth it, because the disease is worse than the treatment." He adds that researchers are working to develop a simpler course of treatment.

Say no to NSAIDs. "Between 15 and 20 percent of people who regularly take NSAIDs have ulcers," reports David Graham, M.D., chief of gastroenterology at the Veterans Adminstration Hospital in Houston. "That's about 20 times the rate in the general population."

If you're taking an NSAID such as aspirin or ibuprofen, Dr. Graham recommends sticking with the lowest possible dose at which the medication is still effective. Or ask your doctor or pharmacist to recommend a substitute. "If you need a pain reliever, for example, there is always Tylenol," Dr. Friedman points out. "The active ingredient is acetaminophen, which doesn't irritate the stomach like NSAIDs do."

Note: Never stop taking a prescription medication without first talking to your doctor.

Try an antacid. "An over-the-counter antacid will provide symptomatic relief," says David Peura, M.D., associate professor of medicine at the University of Virginia Health Sciences Center in Charlottesville. But it is not to be regarded as a cure, he stresses.

Ban the booze. If you're taking antibiotics for your ulcer, refrain from drinking alcoholic beverages during your treatment, advises Dr. Peura. Certain antibiotics can interact with alcohol.

Don't blow smoke. "Studies have shown that smoking is associated with the delayed healing of ulcers," says Naurang Agrawal, M.D., professor of medicine at the University of Connecticut School of Medicine in Farmington.

Take steps to destress. The discovery of *H. pylori* has blurred the relationship between stress and ulcers. One thing is for sure: "Any time you have a chronic condition, stress can make your symptoms worse," Dr. Friedman says. "So it would be wise for anyone with ulcers to learn to manage stress better."

Choose ulcer-friendly fare. Certain foods can aggravate your symptoms. So until your ulcer has healed, "if some food bothers you, avoid it," says Dr. Peura. The usual suspects include spicy cuisine, coffee, and citrus juices.

Also, forget about traditional ulcer remedies such as bland foods and milk. They were never really effective, Dr. Peura says, and now they have fallen out of favor.

Favor fiber. Increasing your intake of dietary fiber with foods such as whole grains and vegetables may help prevent the recurrence of ulcers, says Melvyn Werbach, M.D., a physician in Los Angeles who specializes in nutritional medicine and the author of *Healing with Food.* There is no evidence that fiber can promote the healing of an existing ulcer, he adds.

Go sour on sweets. You may want to cut back on your con sumption of sugar, says Dr. Werbach. "The more refined sugar in your diet, the greater your risk of developing an ulcer—probably because sugar stimulates the secretion of stomach acid," he explains.

Eat earlier. Ulcer patients often wake up in the middle of the night with gnawing pain in their guts. "Researchers have found that the secretion of stomach acid during the night can be reduced by eating dinner earlier in the evening," reports Dr. Werbach. "Less acid secretion should mean less ulcer pain overnight—and perhaps faster healing."

Follow an Eastern path to healing. In Ayurveda, the traditional medical discipline of India, the presence of an ulcer indicates an imbalance of *pitta,* says Brian Rees, M.D., medical director of the Maharishi Ayur-Veda Medical Center in Pacific Palisades, California. Ayurvedic practitioners believe that pitta is one of three basic qualities, or *doshas,* that determine an individual's constitutional body type.

Dr. Rees recommends following a diet that pacifies pitta. That means cutting down on foods with salty, sour, or pungent tastes as well as foods that are fermented or fried.

Varicose Veins

Some people think of varicose veins as nothing more than a cosmetic problem. Yes, those blue bulges and streaks just beneath the surface of the skin may be unsightly. But they're nothing to worry about, right?

Well . . . that all depends. Varicose veins can cause quite a bit of pain. And it's not the sort of pain that just disappears overnight—because varicose veins don't just disappear overnight. Once they show up on your legs (or on your arms, though that's less likely), they're there for the long haul.

A varicose vein forms when the wall of a vein weakens and develops a pocket. In these pockets the blood flow is slowed, leading to inflammation and a dull ache.

Over time, your symptoms can intensify. The area around the vein may become red and tender when you sit or stand for a long period of time. The skin over the vein may become discolored or dry and irritated. The vein itself may ulcerate, which can cause it to bleed.

Since people tend to keep their varicose veins under wraps, you may not realize just how common this condition is. An estimated 30 to 60 percent of adults have them, the majority being women over age 40.

Vanquish Pained Veins

Heredity plays an important part in deciding who gets varicose veins and who doesn't. While you may not be able to stop them from occurring, you can do a lot to ease the discomfort that they cause, says John W. Hallett, M.D., professor of vascular surgery at the Mayo Medical School in Rochester, Minnesota. Here is what he and other doctors recommend to relieve the pain of strained veins.

When to See the Doctor

If you develop varicose veins, you should make your doctor aware of them—regardless of whether they are causing you any discomfort, experts say. Be especially alert for symptoms such as swelling, throbbing, discoloration, and skin breakage, advises Luis Navarro, M.D., director of the Vein Treatment Center in New York City. In such cases, he says, medical treatment is advisable.

Also, you should see your doctor immediately if you experience severe pain, Dr. Navarro says. It may mean that the vein has become infected—a condition known as phlebitis—or that the problem is not with a vein but with a muscle or a bone.

Get a move on. Walk as much as possible, urges Mark Forrestal, M.D., an internist specializing in phlebology and a staff physician at Holy Family Hospital and Christ Hospital in Buffalo Grove, Illinois. "Walking creates a pumping action in your foot and calf, which reduces pressure in the veins on the surface of your legs," he explains. It also helps move the blood back up to your heart so it can't pool in your veins.

Be an opportunist. Take advantage of opportunities during the day to stretch your legs, Dr. Forrestal says. Use the stairs instead of the elevator. Park your car farther from your destination and walk. Instead of sitting and drinking coffee during your break, get up and walk around.

Have a seat when necessary. "Don't sit if you can walk, and don't stand if you can sit," advises Deborah Foley, M.D., an internist at Northwest Community Health Care in Arlington Heights, Illinois. "If you have a job that requires you to stand for long periods of time, try to work it so that you can sit down once in a while." You should also try to walk around for at least 10 minutes every 1½ hours, she says.

Get a leg up. Whenever you are sitting, it's a good idea to elevate your legs, experts agree. "Try to raise them above the level of your heart, if possible," says Luis Navarro, M.D., director of the Vein Treatment Center in New York City.

At night, sleep with your legs on a small incline. "Prop them up on a couple of pillows or elevate the foot end of your bed with some books or bricks," Dr. Navarro suggests. This helps reduce any swelling, which occurs when fluid accumulates in your legs over the course of a day, he explains.

Stock up on support. Support stockings compress the vein and help keep pain and inflammation in check. "They provide varying degrees of pressure," Dr. Navarro explains. "Generally, the more severe the varicose vein, the more pressure that's required." You can buy the stockings over the counter to start, but eventually, your doctor may have to write you a prescription for an even stronger pair. You should wear your stockings for all your waking hours, then take them off while you sleep, he says.

Favor snug-fitting footwear. Your shoes can provide an extra measure of support in the foot and ankle area, which is just where you need it, Dr. Foley says. "You want the highest level of compression at the lowest part of your body," she notes. Just be sure your shoes aren't so snug that they actually make your feet hurt.

Shed some pounds. Overweight doesn't cause varicose veins, but it can definitely aggravate them, experts say. For one thing, it puts extra pressure on your legs—just what strained veins don't need. For another, it's usually a sign of inactivity—too much sitting or standing and not enough moving around, Dr. Forrestal says.

Stay regular. "Straining to move your bowels can affect the valves in the veins of your legs," Dr. Navarro says. When a valve doesn't function properly, it causes the vein wall to weaken, which sets the stage for a varicose vein. If you're prone to constipation, increase your fiber intake, Dr. Navarro suggests. Among the best food sources are fruits, vegetables, and whole-grain breads and cereals.

Give up those garters. Anything that restricts blood circulation to the legs, such as garters, can make vein problems worse, experts say. "Panty hose are okay, though, because they compress the entire leg and help the blood flow toward the heart," Dr. Navarro adds.

Pack some pills. If you're planning a trip by airplane or automobile, you may want to take along some aspirin, Dr. Navarro says. Aspirin has blood-thinning properties, which will counteract the effects of sitting for long periods with your knees bent. He suggests taking one or two tablets 12 to 24 hours before you leave, then continuing at this dosage throughout your trip.

Evaluate estrogen. If you're a woman with a family history of varicose veins, taking birth control pills or hormone replacement therapy may increase your odds of developing the condition, Dr. Navarro says. "Both contain estrogen, and estrogen opens certain connections between arteries and veins, increasing pressure," he explains. You may want to discuss your options with your doctor, he adds.

Windburn

A brisk walk in the wintry air brightens your cheeks with a healthy glow. But add wind to the mix, and that healthy glow may become a raging inferno of redness, swelling, and downright pain.

It's called windburn—which, truth be told, is a misnomer. Yes, it looks like a burn. And it certainly feels like a burn. But it's really a drying effect. "Windburn results from a combination of cold wind and low humidity, which depletes the oil layer on your skin," explains Steven Earl Prawer, M.D., clinical associate professor of dermatology at the University of Minnesota Medical School in Minneapolis.

"It works like a hand dryer in a public bathroom," adds Rodney Basler, M.D., a dermatologist in private practice in Lincoln, Nebraska. "It blows the moisture out of your skin. By dehydrating that outer layer, it ultimately causes inflammation."

As you might have guessed, folks who live in warm southern climates are virtually immune to windburn, unless they take a trip north in the dead of winter. The condition is most likely to affect those who spend time outside in cold, dry, windy weather. And keep in mind that any exposed, unprotected part of your body is vulnerable—not just your face.

Easing the Burn Is a Breeze

A windburn can hurt just as much as a sunburn—but fortunately, it's far less serious. It will usually fade away on its own in a couple of days, provided you take proper care of the affected skin. Here is what the experts recommend to speed the healing process—and to save your skin from future assaults.

When to See the Doctor

Ordinary windburn seldom requires a doctor's care. Symptoms usually disappear on their own within a few days. You should see your doctor, however, if you notice any sign of infection such as crusting, scaling, or oozing, advises David Margolis, M.D., assistant professor of dermatology at the University of Pennsylvania Medical Center in Philadelphia.

If your skin turns very white or starts to blister and you have a lot of pain, seek medical attention at once, Dr. Margolis adds. You may have frostbite.

Hide your hide. It may seem obvious, but your first step should be to get out of the wind, says Dr. Prawer. If you can't escape it, then at least block it any way you can.

Stay moist. Be sure to moisturize windburned skin frequently—perhaps three or four times a day, says David Margolis, M.D., assistant professor of dermatology at the University of Pennsylvania Medical Center in Philadelphia. "The best moisturizer is petroleum jelly, but most people don't find it cosmetically pleasing," he says. "Choose a product that you're comfortable with, as long as it isn't highly scented." Fragrances can cause skin irritations.

Dr. Prawer recommends a thick cream (such as Eucerin). Or follow this two-step procedure suggested by Dr. Basler: Rub 1 percent hydrocortisone cream or ointment on the affected area, then apply Eucerin on top of that.

Pop a pill for the pain. Aspirin will ease any soreness and discomfort associated with windburn, says Dr. Basler. And because it's an anti-inflammatory, it will help speed the healing process as well.

Put your best face forward. If you know you're going to be spending time outside in conditions that produce windburn, then don't wash your face or shave beforehand, advises Dr. Basler. "Doing so removes your skin's natural oils, which offer protection against the environment," he explains.

Don't forget your sunscreen. Just because it's not swimsuit weather doesn't mean that you can't get a sunburn. "The sun is often a factor in complaints of windburn," Dr. Margolis says. He recommends wearing a moisturizer and a sunscreen on days that you're out in cold, dry, windy weather. Look for a product with a sun protection factor (SPF) of at least 15.

Lay it on your kisser. Your lips are especially vulnerable to windburn. Make sure you give them extra protection. Dr. Basler suggests using a lip balm with sunscreen (such as Blistex or Chap Stick).

Don't stick out your neck. "The most vulnerable square inch on your body is the front part of your neck," Dr. Basler says. "The skin there is very thin, and it doesn't get much protection."

Dr. Basler suggests wrapping a terry-cloth towel around your neck. It's actually much better than a wool scarf, he notes: "Wool is irritating to the skin, especially if you're sweating. A towel is much less irritating and more absorbent." You can also wear a turtleneck, of course. Just make sure it's made from cotton, not wool or a synthetic fabric, he says.

Bundle up. When you head outdoors in wintry weather, every exposed part of your body needs to be covered. "Wear gloves to protect your hands and a stocking cap or hood to protect your ears," Dr. Basler says. "Better yet, cover your entire head with a ski mask."

Wrist Pain

The wrist may be the most underappreciated part of the human anatomy. It's so much more than just a convenient place to strap a watch. In fact, the hand couldn't make a move without it.

Within the wrist lies a delicate network of bones, nerves, tendons, and ligaments that supports the hand and controls its actions. Your wrists make it possible for you to perform even the most routine tasks, such as writing a grocery list, tying your shoes, opening a jar, and waving good-bye.

You may not realize just how important your wrists are until one of them gets hurt. "There are basically two types of wrist injury," says Joel Press, M.D., associate professor of clinical physical medicine and rehabilitation at Northwestern University Medical School in Chicago. "One is acute, such as a sprain or a fracture. The other is overuse, caused by the repetitive motion of activities such as typing."

The overuse injury that most often affects the wrists is tendinitis. "The tendons responsible for the movement of the fingers and hand get inflamed—especially around the thumb and little finger," explains John Cianca, M.D., assistant professor of physical medicine and rehabilitation at the Baylor College of Medicine in Houston. "People who use their hands a lot—carpenters, computer operators, musicians—can develop tendinitis if the tendons in their wrists aren't strong and flexible enough."

Overuse can also affect the ulnar nerve, which runs along the pinkie side of the wrist and hand. And it can cause tissues in the wrist to swell and put pressure on the median nerve, leading to carpal tunnel syndrome. Both conditions can produce tingling, numbness, and pain in the fingers and hands as well as in the wrists. (To find out more about carpal tunnel syndrome, see the chapter on page 51.)

Watch Those Wrists

No matter what its cause, wrist pain will certainly grab your attention. How can you get relief? Here's what the experts recommend.

Give it a rest. The best thing you can do for an aching wrist is use it as little as possible, says Edward A. Rankin, M.D., chief of orthopedic surgery at Providence Hospital in Washington, D.C. "Resting your wrist will allow any swelling to go down," he explains.

Break it up. If you must use your wrist, Dr. Cianca recommends taking frequent breaks from repetitive tasks. "Instead of typing for an hour straight, for example, type for 15 minutes and then rest your wrist for a bit," he says.

Put it on the rocks. "Ice is a vasoconstrictor," Dr. Rankin says. "That means it decreases the blood supply in your wrist, which helps reduce any swelling." He suggests putting ice cubes in a plastic bag, wrapping the bag in a towel, and applying the pack to your wrist for about 20 minutes. Repeat the treatment four to six times a day, he adds.

Turn on the heat. Once any swelling subsides—or if your wrist simply feels stiff and achy—heat can help, says Arthur H. Brownstein, M.D., a physician in Princeville, Hawaii, and clinical instructor of medicine at the University of Hawaii School of Medicine in Manoa. His instructions: Rub vinegar on your wrist, cover it with plastic, then apply a heating pad (wrapped in a towel) for about 20 minutes. You can repeat this treatment every hour as needed.

Treat it gingerly. A compress made from ginger can draw out toxins and accelerate the healing process, Dr. Brownstein says. To make the compress, simply boil some grated gingerroot, allow it to cool, place it in a moist washcloth, and lay the washcloth over your wrist. The washcloth should be as hot as you can tolerate, he notes. Leave it on for 15 to 20 minutes, and repeat every other hour.

Raise your hand. Elevation is not as crucial for an injured wrist as for an injured ankle or knee, Dr. Press says. Still, it can help

When to See the Doctor

If you sustain an acute wrist injury such as a fracture or a sprain, you should get proper medical care right away, says Joel Press, M.D., associate professor of clinical physical medicine and rehabilitation at Northwestern University Medical School in Chicago. Wrist pain that lasts for more than a few days also warrants a doctor's attention—especially if it is limiting your activity, if it disrupts your sleep, or if it is accompanied by swelling.

keep any swelling down. "Just be sure to prop your wrist so that it's above heart level," he advises.

Don't be a leaner. Leaning on your elbows—when you sit at a desk, for example—can worsen wrist pain, says Ed Laskowski, M.D., co-director of the Sportsmedicine Center at the Mayo Clinic in Rochester, Minnesota. It puts pressure on the ulnar nerve, which runs all the way down your arm into your wrist and hand.

Keep still. For a more severe case of tendinitis, immobilizing the joint with an elastic wrist support (also called a wrist splint) may provide some relief, Dr. Rankin says. You'll find these devices in drugstores and medical supply stores. He suggests wearing one while you sleep—to prevent your wrist from twisting awkwardly—as well as during your waking hours, when your wrist is in use. "The support should keep your wrist in about a 10-degree dorsiflex position," he advises. In other words, if your palm is facing downward, your wrist should be bent slightly upward.

Note: Do not wear a wrist support to treat a severe sprain or fracture, Dr. Press advises. See your doctor instead.

Opt for over-the-counter relief. A nonsteroidal anti-inflammatory drug (NSAID) such as ibuprofen or naproxen (Aleve) can ease your discomfort, experts say. Choose the one that works best for you. "Patients have individual responses to these drugs," Dr. Rankin notes.

Ease back into it. A wrist that has been immobilized may become stiff from lack of use, Dr. Brownstein notes. Some gentle stretching can help restore flexibility.

Dr. Brownstein suggests pressing on a tabletop with the palm of your hand. "Bend your wrist until you reach the angle of pain, then back off just a hair," he says. "By riding the edge of discomfort and stopping just before you feel pain, you're doing beneficial stretching." Hold this position for as long as you find comfortable, working up to 2 minutes. Repeat three to four times daily.

Build some muscle. You can prevent future wrist pain by strengthening the muscles in your forearms, Dr. Cianca says. He recommends holding a 6-ounce can of tomato paste in each hand and flexing your wrists back and forth 15 to 20 times. Or you can simply squeeze a tennis ball in each hand, he says. Squeeze the ball for 5 seconds and release, then repeat 12 to 15 times.

Index

Boldfaced page references indicate main discussion of topic and "When to See the Doctor" boxes. Underscored page references indicate boxed text.

A

Abscesses, rectal, **98–100, 99**
Acetaminophen in relieving
  bedsores, 17
  headache, 128
  hip pain, 143
  knee pain, 162
  penile pain, 192
  phantom limb, 195
  shingles, 217
  sore throat, 237
  toothache, 276
Acid inhibitors, 131, 245–46
Acidophilus, canker sores and, 49–50
Acid reflux, 133
Acupressure in relieving
  neck pain, 186
  toothache, 276
Acupuncture in relieving
  cancer pain, 46
  facial pain, 97
  penile pain, 192
  postoperative pain, 202
  testicular pain, 267
Acuscope, phantom limb and, 196
Acyclovir (Rx), 111, <u>216</u>
Additives, food, 95, 172
Airplane ear, 78, 81–82
Alcohol
  absorption of, 123
  dehydration and, 124–25
  exercise and, 229
  gout and, 114–16
  hangover, 123–25, **124**
  kidney stones and, 159
  migraine and, 173

  side stitches and, 229
  ulcers and, 280
Aleve. *See* Naproxen in relieving
Allergies, 48–49, 238
Aloe vera in relieving
  burns, 34
  cancer pain, from injections, 46
  cuts and scrapes, 70
American Academy of Head and Facial
  Pain, **80**
American Cancer Society's national
  resource center, <u>47</u>
American Dental Association, **277**
American Pain Society, <u>47</u>
American Society for Clinical Hypnosis, 46
Amputation, pain from, **193–98, 194**, <u>195</u>
Analgesics. *See specific types*
Anger, stomach pain and, 246–47
Angina, **1–3, 3**
Ankle pain, **4–6, 5**
Antacids in relieving
  canker sores, 49
  chemical burns, 35
  heartburn, 131
  stomach pain, 245
  ulcer symptoms, 280
Antibiotics, 267
Anticonvulsants, 196
Antidepressants, 196, <u>216</u>
Antidiarrheal medications, 246
Antigas medications, 110
Antihistamines, sinus pain and, 230
Antioxidants, genital herpes and, 113
Antiseizure drugs, postherpetic neuralgia
  and, <u>216</u>
Anxiety, stomach pain and, 246

Apis remedy, eye pain and, 90
Appendicitis, stomach pain and, 242
Arachidonic acid in red meat, 85
Arches, high or fallen, 22, **40**, 162, 221
Arch supports, 32, 42
Arginine, cold sores and, 62
Arnica, bursitis and, 37
Aromatherapy. *See specific essential oils*
Arthritis, **7–10**, **8**, 141
Artificial sweeteners, migraine and, 172
Artificial tears, eye lubrication and, 65, 89
Aspartame, migraine and, 172
Aspirin
   as blood thinner, 267, 285
   in heart attack prevention, 3
   sucking on, avoiding, 122, 237
   in relieving
      bursitis, 37
      endometriosis, 86
      genital herpes, 112
      hangover, 124–25
      headache, 128
      knee pain, 162
      migraine, 175
      muscle cramps, 179
      penile pain, 192
      phantom limb, 195
      sunburn, 252
      temporomandibular disorder, 259
      tennis elbow, 263
      windburn, 287
Attitude, postoperative pain and, 201
Aura in migraine, 170

B

Baby oil
   ear pain and, 79
   ingrown toenail and, 148
   swimmer's ear and, 81
Back pain, **11–16**, 12, **14**
Baclofen (Rx), 196
Baking soda paste in relieving
   canker sores, 49
   chemical burns, 35
   gum pain, 121

Balms. *See* Ointments
Bandages. *See* Dressings
Baths
   foot
      for corns, 66
      Domeboro solution in, 147
      essential oils in, 103, 115
      for foot pain, 103
      for gout, 115
      for ingrown toenail, 147
   paraffin, 9
   sitz
      for fissures and abscesses, rectal, 98
      for hemorrhoids, 138
   splinters and, 241
   sunburn and, 252–53
Beano, 110
Bedsores, **17–18**, **18**
BenGay ointment, calf pain and, 40
Benzocaine, pizza burn and, 198
Beta-carotene, antioxidants in, 113
Betadine iodine preparation, 217
Bic's Original or Sensitive Shaver, 204
Bicycle, stationary, in preventing
   knee pain, 165
   shinsplints, 221
Bile, 105
Biofeedback, migraine and, 174
Biotin, nails and, 29
Birth control pills
   breast pain and, 27
   intercourse pain and, 153
   varicose veins and, 285
Bleeding
   with muscle spasms, **182**
   rectal, **109**
Blisters
   fever, 60–62, **61**
   foot, 20–22, **21**
   genital herpes and, **112**
Blistex, 60, 288
Blood sugar levels, 130, 172
Body fat. *See* Overweight
Bouillon, hangover and, 124
Bra, breast pain and, 25–26

Boldfaced page references indicate main discussion of topic and "When to See the Doctor" boxes. <u>Underscored</u> page references indicate boxed text.

Braces
  knee, 162
  neck, **188**
Breakfast, gallbladder disease and,
  107
Breast pain, **23–27**, <u>24</u>, **26**
Breathing technique, proper, for side
  stitches, 228
Broken nails, **28–29**, **29**, 250
Bromelain, shinsplints and, 220
Brushing teeth, 119
Bunions, **30–32**, **31**
Burning tongue syndrome, <u>270–71</u>
Burns, **33–35**, **34**
Bursae, 36
Bursitis, **36–38**, **38**
B vitamins. *See also specific types*
  deficiency in, 272
  endometriosis and, 85

C

Caffeine
  breast pain and, 25
  gout pain and, 116
  headache and, 128–29, <u>129</u>
  irritable bowel syndrome and, 156
  kidney stones and, 159
  migraine and, 172
Calcium
  in osteoporosis prevention, <u>142</u>
  kidney stones and, 160
Calcium kidney stones, 158
Calf pain, **39–42**, **40**
Calluses, foot, **31**
Cancer
  mouth, **73**
  prostate, 190
  skin, 251
Cancer pain, **43–47**, <u>44</u>, <u>45</u>, <u>47</u>
Cane, walking with, 143, 164
Canker sores, **48–50**, **49**
Capsaicin in ointments, 8–9, 97, <u>216</u>
Carbamazepine (Rx), <u>216</u>
Carbohydrates, irritable bowel syndrome
  and, 156

Carpal tunnel syndrome (CTS), **51–53**,
  52, 289
Castor-oil pack, endometriosis pain and,
  84
Cetaphil soap
  chafing and, 55
  sunburn and, 252
Chafing, **54–56**, **55**
Chap Stick, 288
Checkups. *See* Examinations
Chemical burn, 35
Chemotherapy, cancer pain and, 43
Chicken pox virus, 215, 218
Childbirth classes, 57–58
Childbirth pain, **57–59**, **58**
Chlorhexidine rinse, gum pain and,
  121–22
Cholesterol levels, 2, 105, 113
Circulatory problems, 146, **148**
Citrucel, as fiber supplement, 155
Clothing
  chafing and, 55
  shingles and, 218
  sunburn and, 253
  windburn and, 288
Cluster headache, 126
Codeine (Rx), 100
Coffee. *See* Caffeine
Colds, 235
Cold compress in relieving
  burn pain, 33
  genital herpes, 111
  migraine, 171
  shingles, 217
  sunburn, 251–52
  temporomandibular disorder, 256
Cold sores, **60–62**, **61**
Colloidal silver in relieving
  genital herpes sores, 112
  shingles blisters, 217
Compression. *See* Wraps
Computers
  eyestrain and, <u>93</u>
  neck pain and, 187
  repetitive strain injury and, 207

Boldfaced page references indicate main discussion of topic and "When to See the
Doctor" boxes. <u>Underscored</u> page references indicate boxed text.

Conjunctivitis, 89–90
Constipation
    enema in relieving, 99
    fiber and, 284
    fissures and abscesses and, rectal, 99
    from medications, 100, 201
Contraceptives, oral. *See* Birth control
        pills
Corneal burns and abrasions, **63–65**, **64**
Corns, **66–68**, **68**
Coronary arteries, blocked, 1–2
Corset, back pain and, 13
Corticosteroids, carpal tunnel syndrome
        and, **42**
Cracked tooth, 273
Cramps, muscle, **176–80**, **177**
Creams. *See* Ointments
Crutches, walking with, 143, 164
CTS, **51–53**, **52**, 289
Cubital tunnel syndrome, 262
Cupping technique, eyestrain and, 92
Cushion, heel, 137
Cuts and scrapes, **69–71**, 70, **71**

D

Dairy foods. *See also* Milk products
    endometriosis and, 85
    gas pain and, 108–9
    irritable bowel syndrome and, 155
    stomach pain and, 244
Danazol (Rx), 86
Danocrine (Rx), 86
Decay, tooth, 273
Decongestants
    airplane ear and, 81–82
    sinus pain and, 230–31
Deep breathing
    childbirth and, 58–59
    headache and, 128
Dehydration, 123–25, 159, 229
Dental care, **118**, 119, 272
Dental problems. *See* Mouth problems
Denture pain, **72–74**, **73**
De-pressurizing devices, bedsores and,
        18–19

Detergents, laundry, chafing and, 56
Diabetes, 146, **148**
Diamox (Rx), 175
Diarrhea
    evening primrose oil and, 27
    medications, 246
    with stomach pain, 246
    from vitamin C overload, 125, 180,
        259
Diet. *See also* Eating habits; Food
    breast pain and, 23–25
    denture pain and, 72–73
    migraine and, 172
    side stitches and, 229
    sodium-rich, 158
    stomach pain and, 243
Dietary fat
    arthritis and, 9
    breast pain and, 25
    gallbladder pain and, 105–6
    kidney stones and, 158
Dieting, 106
Digestive problems
    constipation, 99–100, 201, 284
    diarrhea, 27, 125, 180, 246, 259
    diverticulitis and, 75–76, **76**
    diverticulosis, 75–77, **76**
    gallbladder pain, 105–7, **106**
    gas pain, 108–10, **109**
    hunger pangs, 243
    irritable bowel syndrome, 154–56, **155**
    stomach pain, 242–47, **244**
    ulcers, stomach, 278–81, **279**
Disk
    herniated, 210
    ruptured, 185
Dislocation of hip, 141
Diverticulitis, 75–76, **76**
Diverticulosis, **75–77**, **76**
DL phenylalanine, menstrual pain and,
        168
Docusate sodium in stool softeners, 99
Domeboro solution, foot baths and, 147
Doshas, in Ayurveda, 281
Doxidan, 99

Boldfaced page references indicate main discussion of topic and "When to See the Doctor" boxes. Underscored page references indicate boxed text.

Dressings
    for bedsores, 17
    for blisters, 20
    for broken nails, 28
    for burns, 34–35
    for chafing, 54–55
    for cuts and scrapes, 70, <u>70</u>
Drugs. *See* Medications; *specific types*
Dry eye, 87

E

Earache, 78
Ear pain, **77–82**, **80**
Eating habits. See also Diet
    exercise and, 228–29
    gas pain and, 109
    headache and, 130
    heartburn and, 132
    irritable bowel syndrome and, 156
    overeating, avoiding, 245
    relaxation during meals and, 77
    time of meals and, 2
    ulcers and, 281
Ejaculation pain, <u>152</u>
Elavil (Rx), 196
Electrolytes, muscle contractions and,
    179, **228**
Elevation in relieving
    foot pain, 103
    sinus pain, 232
    sunburn pain, 252
    wrist pain, 290–91
Emotional distress, stomach pain and, 246
Endometriosis, **83–86**, **84**
Endorphins, exercise and, 45, 167
Enema, constipation and, 99
Epididymis, 265
Epididymitis, 265
Epidural, childbirth pain and, **58**
Epsom salts, hemorrhoids and, 138–39
Essential oils, foot baths and, 103, 115
Estrogen
    breast pain and, 27
    migraine and, 173
    varicose veins and, 285

Eustachian tube, 78, 82
Evening primrose oil, breast pain and,
    26
Examinations
    bone mass, <u>142</u>
    dental, **118**, 272
    eye, 94
Exercise. *See also* Physical activity;
    specific types
    after alcohol consumption, 229
    ankle-strengthening, 6
    aquatic, 144, 221
    arm, 208–9
    back-strengthening, 14–15
    biting, for temporomandibular
        disorder, 258, 260
    calf-strengthening, 42, 180
    dehydration and, 159
    diverticular disease and, 77
    after eating, 228–29
    elbow-strengthening, 264
    endometriosis and, 84–85
    endorphins and, 45, 167
    eye, 93
    foot, 104
    hand, 208–9
    hangover and, 124
    heel, 137
    hemorrhoids and, 140
    leg-strengthening, 222
    neck, 189
    pelvic, 211–12
    piriformis muscle, 213
    postoperative pain and, 201
    in preventing
        fractures, <u>142</u>
        heart attack, 3
    range-of-motion, 37–38, 225
    in relieving
        arthritis pain, 8
        cancer pain, 45
    shinsplints and, 222
    shoulder, 37–38, 189, 208, 225–26
    stretching, 144–45, <u>178</u>, 225
    thigh-strengthening, 164

Boldfaced page references indicate main discussion of topic and "When to See the Doctor" boxes. <u>Underscored</u> page references indicate boxed text.

Exercise *(continued)*
  visualization, 45
  wrist, 208–9, 292
Ex-Lax stool softener, 99
Extra Strength Tylenol, 80
Eye pain, **87–90**, **88**
Eye problems
  conjunctivitis, 89–90
  corneal burns and abrasions, 63–65, **64**
  dry eye, 87
  glaucoma, **88**
  injury, 88
  pain, 87–90, **88**
  strain, 91–94, **92**, 93
  sty, 89–90
Eyestrain, **91–94**, **92**, 93

F

Facial pain, **94–97**, **96**
Famciclovir (Rx), 111
Famvir (Rx), 111
Fat. *See* Dietary fat; Overweight
Fennel tea, gas pain and, 109
Fenugreek, menstrual pain and, 168–69
Fever blisters, 60–62, **61**
Fiber
  constipation and, 284
  diverticulosis and, 75–76
  fissures and abscesses and, rectal, 100
  gas pain and, 109
  hemorrhoids and, 140
  irritable bowel syndrome and, 155–56
  supplements, 155
  ulcers and, 281
Fish, omega-3 fatty acids in, 9, 85, 174
Fissures, rectal, **98–100**, **99**
Flexibility
  arm and shoulder, 226
  joint, 8
  muscle, 183–84
Flossing teeth, 119
Fluid intake
  diverticulosis and, 77
  endometriosis and, 85
  fissures and abscesses and, rectal, 100

hangover and, 125
heartburn and, 132
hemorrhoids and, 139
kidney stones and, 158
muscle cramps and, 179
side stitches and, 229
sinus pain and, 231–32
sore throat and, 235
sports drinks and, 123–24, 179
stomach pain and, 245
Fluid retention, 25
Flushes. *See* Rinses
Food. *See also* Diet; *specific types*
  additives, 95, 172
  allergies, 48–49
  canker sores and, 48–49
  chewing, 257
  diary, 154–55, 172, 247
  gas-producing, 108
  gum pain and, 121
  migraine and, 172
  oxalate-rich, 159
  pizza burn and, 198
  protein-rich, 125
  purine-rich, 114–15
  raffinose in, 110
  seeds in, 76–77
  sore throat and, 238
  stomach pain and, 243
  sugary, 167
  temporomandibular disorder and, 256
  tongue pain and, 269
  toothache and, 275
  ulcers and, 281
Foot care, 21
Foot pain, **101–4**, 102, **103**
Foot problems
  ankle pain, 4–6, **5**
  blisters, 20–22, **21**
  bunions, 30–32, **31**
  calluses, **31**
  corns, 66–68, **68**
  heel pain, 134–37, 135, **136**
  ingrown toenail, 146–49, 147, **148**

pain, 101–4, <u>102</u>, **103**
plantar fasciitis, 137
stubbed toe, 248–50, **249**
Fractures
chip, **38**
penile, <u>191</u>
preventing, <u>142</u>
toe, 248
Frozen shoulder, 36, 224
Fructose, alcohol absorption and, 123

G

Gallbladder pain, **105–7, 106**
Gallstones, 105
Gargling, 237
Garlic, ear pain and, 79
Garters, varicose veins and, 284–85
Gas pain, **108–10, 109**
Gastroesophageal reflux, **131–33, 132,**
<u>235</u>
Gatorade, 123–24, 179
Genital herpes, **111–13, 112**
Ginger compresses
ankle pain and, 5
tennis elbow and, 262
wrist pain and, 290
Gingivitis, 117, 121–22
Glaucoma, **88**
Glycerine, 237
GnRH agonists, endometriosis and, 86
Goldenseal powder, cancer pain and,
46
Gout, **114–16, 115**
Grinding, tooth, 258
Gum pain, **117–22, 118,** <u>120–21</u>

H

Hair dryer, swimmer's ear and, 81
Hallux valgus, **30–32, 31**
Hangover, **123–25, 124**
HDL, 2
Headache, **126–30, 127,** <u>129</u>
Heart attack prevention, 2–3
Heartburn, **131–33, 132, 279**
Heart problems, **1–3, 3**

Heat in relieving
ankle pain, 5
arthritis, **7–8**
back pain, 12–13
endometriosis, 84
eyestrain, 92
facial pain, 97
headache, 127
heel pain, 136
hip pain, 143
menstrual pain, 167
muscle cramps, 179
muscle spasms, 182–83
penile pain, 191
postoperative pain, 200
shinsplints, 221
shoulder pain, 225
stubbed toe, 249
temporomandibular disorder, 256
tennis elbow, 262
wrist pain, 290
Heel pain, **134–37,** <u>135</u>, **136**
Heel-raiser, 137
Helicobacter pylori, 278–80
Hemorrhoids, 98, **138–40, 139**
Herbal therapy. *See specific herbs*
Heredity, varicose veins and, 282
Herpes simplex type 2, **111–13, 112**
Herpes zoster, **215–18,** <u>216</u>, **218**
High blood pressure, 3
High-density lipoprotein (HDL), 2
Hip pain, **141–45,** <u>142</u>, **144**
Hoku pressure point, toothache and, 276
Homeopathy. *See specific remedies*
Honey
alcohol absorption and, 123
tea with, sore throat and, 236–37
Hormone replacement therapy, breast pain
and, 27
Housemaid's knee, 161
Humidifier, sore throat and, 236
Hunger pangs, 243
Hydantoin (Rx), <u>216</u>
Hydration, **228**
Hydrochloric acid deficiency, 107

Boldfaced page references indicate main discussion of topic and "When to See the Doctor" boxes. Underscored page references indicate boxed text.

Hydrocollator, arthritis and, 10
Hydrocortisone cream, sunburn and, 252
Hydrogen peroxide, gum pain and, 119–21, _120_
Hygiene
  cold sores and, 62
  fissures and abscesses and, rectal, 99
  gingivitis and, 117
  hemorrhoids and, 139
  oral, 117, 119
  shingles and, 217
Hypersensitivity, dental, 273
Hypertension, 3
Hypnosis
  cancer pain and, 46
  childbirth pain and, 59

I

IBS, **154–56**, **155**
Ibuprofen in relieving
  ankle pain, 6
  back pain, 13
  breast pain, 27
  bunion pain, 32
  calf pain, 40–41
  endometriosis, 86
  genital herpes, 112
  hangovers, 125
  headache, 128
  heel pain, 136
  hip pain, 143
  ingrown toenail, 148
  knee pain, 162
  menstrual pain, 169
  muscle spasms, 183
  phantom limb, 195
  pizza burn, 198
  postoperative pain, 201–2
  shoulder pain, 225
  sore throat, 237
  sunburn, 252
  tennis elbow, 263
  wrist pain, 291

Ice in relieving
  arthritis, 7
  back pain, 11–12
  bunions, 30
  bursitis, 36–37
  carpal tunnel syndrome, 52
  cold sores, 60
  dry eyes, 89
  facial pain, 96–97
  foot pain, 103
  gout, 115
  headache, 127
  heel pain, 136
  hip pain, 141, 143
  knee pain, 162
  muscle cramps, 179
  muscle spasms, 182
  penile pain, 191–92
  postoperative pain, 200
  shinsplints, 221
  shoulder pain, 225
  splinters, 239
  stubbed toe, 249
  tennis elbow, 261
  testicular pain, 265–66
  wrist pain, 290
Imitrex (Rx), _173_
Imodium, 246
Indigestion, **131–33**, **132**, **279**
Infection
  ear, 79, 81
  eyelid, 89–90
  middle-ear, 78
  signs of, **71**, 217
  sinus, _274_
  yeast, _271_
Ingrown toenail, **146–49**, _147_, **148**
Intercourse pain, **150–53**, **151**, _152_
Intermittent claudication, 39, **40**
Intravenous medications, cancer pain and, 46–47
Iodine preparation, shingles and, 217
Iron deficiency, _270_
Irritable bowel syndrome (IBS), **154–56**, **155**

Boldfaced page references indicate main discussion of topic and "When to See the Doctor" boxes. Underscored page references indicate boxed text.

J

Jaw problems, **73**, 78, 95, 255–60, <u>257</u>, **259**
Joint problems
    arthritis, 7–10, **8**, 141
    bursitis, 36–38, **38**
    gout, 114–16, **115**
    tendinitis, **38**, 291
Juniper, foot baths and, 103, 115

K

Kidney stones, **157–60, 158**
Knee pain, **161–65, 163**
Krazy Glue, paper cuts and, 70
K-Y Jelly, vaginal dryness and, 151

L

Labor pain, **57–59, 58**
Lactaid, 155
Lactic acid, 124
Lactose
    intolerance, 109, 153, 244
    migraine and, 172
    stomach pain and, 244
Lamaze method of childbirth, 57
Laparoscopic surgery, 86
Lateral epicondylitis, **261–64**, <u>262</u>, **263**
Lavender, foot baths and, 103
LDL, 2
Leg problems
    calf pain, 39–42, **40**
    hip pain, 141–45, <u>142</u>, **144**
    intermittent claudication, 39, **40**
    knee pain, **161–65, 163**
    muscle cramps, 176–80, **177**
    phlebitis, 39, **40**
    shinsplints, 219–22, <u>220</u>, **222**
    varicose veins, 282–85, **283**
Lidocaine viscous, tongue pain and, 271
Lifting technique, heavy, <u>12</u>, 224
Lifts, heel, 41
Lighting, eyestrain and, 94
Limping, 164
Lip balm
    cold sores and, 60
    windburn and, 288

Listerine mouthwash, gum pain and, 122
Locked jaw, <u>257</u>
Low-density lipoprotein (LDL), 2
Lozenges, throat
    menthol, 237
    mint in, 237
    sorbitol in, 74
    sore throat and, 237
Lubrication, intercourse pain and, 151
Lysine
    cold sores and, 61
    genital herpes and, 113
    supplements, 61

M

Magnesia phosphorica, menstrual pain
    and, 167–68
Magnesium levels, 174
Makeup application, temporomandibular
    disorder and, 258
Mammogram, <u>24</u>
Massage in relieving
    breast pain, 25
    bursitis, 37
    cancer pain, 46
    denture pain, 73
    eyestrain, 92
    facial pain, 96–97
    foot pain, 104
    muscle cramps, 179
    muscle spasms, 183
    neck pain, 186
    phantom limb, 194
    shinsplints, 221
Mastalgia, **23–27**, <u>24</u>, **26**
Maxillary sinusitis, <u>274</u>
Meat, red
    arachidonic acid in, 85
    diverticulosis and, 77
    endometriosis and, 85
    kidney stones and, 158
Medial epicondylitis, <u>262</u>
Medications. *See also specific types*
    angina, 1–2
    antidiarrheal, 246

Boldfaced page references indicate main discussion of topic and "When to See the Doctor" boxes. <u>Underscored</u> page references indicate boxed text.

Medications *(continued)*
 antigas, 110
 effects of
  burning tongue syndrome, 270–71
  constipation, 100, 201
  dry mouth, 74
  heartburn, 133
  uric acid increase, 116
 intravenous, for cancer pain, 46–47
 metabolism of, 44
Menopause, 270
Menstrual pain, **166–69**, **168**
Menstruation, **24**, 83, **84**, 175
Menthol lozenges, 237
Metabolism
 of cholesterol, 105
 headache and, 129
 of medications, 44
Metamucil, as fiber supplement, 155
Metatarsal joint, stubbed toe and, 248
Methylcellulose in fiber supplements, 155
Middle-ear infection, 78
Midwife, childbirth pain and, 59
Migraine, 126, **170–75**, **171**, 173
Milk products. *See also* Dairy foods
 gas pain and, 109
 irritable bowel syndrome and, 155
 kidney stones and, 160
 lactose intolerance and, 109, 153, 244
Mineral oil
 ear pain and, 79
 swimmer's ear and, 81
Minerals. *See specific types*
Mint in lozenges, 237
Moisturizers
 broken nails and, 29
 razor burn and, 205
 windburn and, 287
Moleskin patch, blisters and, 21
Monosodium glutamate (MSG)
 facial pain and, 95
 migraine and, 172
Mouth-care products, 271
Mouthpiece, temporomandibular disorder
  and, 258–59

Mouth problems
 burning tongue syndrome, 270–71
 canker sores, 48–50, **49**
 cold sores, 60–62, **61**
 cracked tooth, 273
 decayed tooth, 273
 denture pain, 72–74, **73**
 gingivitis, 117, 121–22
 grinding teeth, 258
 gum pain, 117–22, **118**, 120–21
 hypersensitivity, dental, 273
 pizza burn, 197–98, **198**
 tongue pain, 268–72, **269**, 270–71
 toothache, 273–77, 274, **277**
MSG. *See* Monosodium glutamate
Muscle problems
 cramps, 176–80, **177**
 repetitive strain injury, 206–9, **208**
 shinsplints, 219–22, 220, **222**
 side stitches, 227–29, **228**
 spasms, 181–84, **182**

N
Nails, broken, **28–29**, **29**, 250
Nail-trimming technique, 149
Naproxen in relieving
 ingrown toenail, 148
 knee pain, 162
 menstrual pain, 169
 pizza burn, 198
 wrist pain, 291
Narcotics (Rx), 216. *See also specific types*
Nasal spray, airplane ear and, 81–82
Nausea, 243
Neck pain, **185–89**, **187**, 188
Neosporin ointment
 chafing and, 54
 penile abrasions and, 192
Nerve blocks, regional, phantom limb and,
  194
Neuroma pain, 195
Niacin deficiency, 270
Nicotine. *See* Smoking
Nitrates, migraine and, 172
Nitroglycerin (Rx), 1–2

Boldfaced page references indicate main discussion of topic and "When to See the Doctor" boxes. Underscored page references indicate boxed text.

Nonsteroidal anti-inflammatory drugs
    (NSAIDs)
  effects of
    heartburn, 133
    ulcers, 278, 280
  in relieving
    ankle pain, 6
    back pain, 13
    breast pain, 27
    bunions, 32
    bursitis, 37
    calf pain, 40–41
    endometriosis, 86
    facial pain, 97
    genital herpes, 112
    heel pain, 136
    ingrown toenails, 147–48
    menstrual pain, 169
    migraines, _173_
    muscle spasms, 183
    neck pain, 186
    pizza burn, 198
    postoperative pain, 201–2
    sciatica pain, 211
    shingles, 217
    shoulder pain, 225
    temporomandibular disorder, 259
    tennis elbow, 263
    toothache, 276
    wrist pain, 291
Nurse-midwives, childbirth pain and, 59
NutraSweet, migraine and, 172
Nutrition. _See_ Diet

O

Oilatum soap, sunburn and, 253
Oil of cloves, toothache and, 275–76
Oils. _See specific types_
Ointments
  capsaicin in, 8–9, 97, _216_
  natural progesterone, 85–86, 169
  in preventing
    blisters, 21
    broken nails, 29
    windburn, 288

  in relieving
    arthritis, 8–9
    burns, 34
    calf pain, 40
    chafing, 54
    cold sores, 60–61
    genital herpes, 111–12
    gum pain, _121_
    hemorrhoids, 138–39
    penile abrasions, 192
    pizza burn, 198
    razor burn, 204
    sunburn, 252–53
    trigeminal neuralgia, 97
  yam-derived, 86, 169
Olive oil, ingrown toenail and, 148
Omega-3 fatty acids, 9, 85, 174
Onycholysis, _147_
Orajel
  canker sores and, 50
  denture pain and, 50
  tongue pain and, 271–72
Oral candidiasis, _271_
Orthotics
  bunions and, 31–32
  foot pain and, 104
Osteoarthritis, 7
OTC drugs. _See specific types_
Otitis media, 78
Overeating, avoiding, 245
Overpronation of foot, 162, 221
Over-the-counter (OTC) drugs. _See_
    specific types
Overweight
  arthritis and, 9
  carpal tunnel syndrome and, 53
  gallbladder pain and, 106
  gout and, 114, 116
  varicose veins and, 284
Oxalate in urine, 159

P

Pads, corn, 66
Paper cuts, 70
Paraffin dips, arthritis pain and, 9

Boldfaced page references indicate main discussion of topic and "When to See the Doctor" boxes. Underscored page references indicate boxed text.

Paronychia, <u>147</u>
Patch, eye, 64
PC muscle, 152–53
Pelvic pain, **84**, **168**
Pelvic tilts, 211–12
Penile pain, <u>152</u>, **190–92**, **191**
Peridex rinse, gum pain and, 122
Periodontitis, 117–18
Person controlled analgesia, cancer pain and, 47
Petroleum jelly
    blisters and, 21
    broken nails and, 29
    cuts and scrapes and, 71
Peyronie's disease, 190, 192
Phantom limb pain, **193–98**, **194**, <u>195</u>
Phenylethylamine, migraine and, 172
Phlebitis, 39, **40**
Physical activity. *See also* Exercise
    back pain and, 15–16
    bedsores and, 18
    headache and, 130
    knee pain and, 162
    sciatica and, 211
Physical therapy in relieving
    phantom limb pain, 196
    tennis elbow, 264
Piles, 138
Piriformis muscle, 213
Pizza burn, **197–98**, **198**
Plantar fasciitis, 137
Plaque, dental, 119, 121–22
Plasters, corn, 67
Postherpetic neuralgia, <u>216</u>
Postoperative pain, **199–202**, **200**
Posture
    back pain and, 13
    for computer work, <u>93</u>
    neck pain and, 185
    for reading, 94
    repetitive strain injury and, 207
Potassium deficiency, 179–80, **228**
Powder, chafing and, 55
Preparation H ointment, 138
Prescription drugs. *See specific types*

Pressure points
    headache and, 128
    migraine and, 172
    temporomandibular disorder and, 260
    toothache and, 276
Priapism, <u>152</u>
ProGest, 85–86
Progesterone, natural, 85–86, 169
Prostaglandins, 85, 167, 169
Prostate gland, <u>152</u>, 190
Prostatitis, 190
Psoriasis, **204**
Psyllium in fiber supplements, 155
Pubococcygeal (PC) muscle, 152–53
Purines in foods, 114–15

R

Raffinose in food, 110
Range-of-motion exercise, 37–38, 225
Razor burn, **203–5**, **204**
Reading, correct posture for, 94
Referred pain, 265
Reflexology, 276–77. *See also* Pressure points
Relaxation techniques
    in preventing
        heart attack, 3
        migraine, 173–74
        ulcers, 280–81
    in relieving
        arthritis, 9
        bedsores, 9
        breast pain, 26
        cancer pain, 45–46
        childbirth, 58–59
        cold sores, 62
        facial pain, 97
        genital herpes, 113
        headache, 129
        irritable bowel syndrome, 156
        menstrual pain, 167
        phantom limb, 195
        shingles, <u>216</u>
        temporomandibular disorder, 260
Repetitive strain injury, **206–9**, **208**

Boldfaced page references indicate main discussion of topic and "When to See the Doctor" boxes. <u>Underscored</u> page references indicate boxed text.

Replens, 151
Reproductive problems
  endometriosis, 83–86, **84**
  epididymitis, 265
  genital herpes, 111–13, **112**
  intercourse pain, 150–53, **151**, <u>152</u>
  menstrual pain, 166–69, **168**
  penile pain, <u>152</u>, 190–92, **191**
  Peyronie's disease, 190, 192
  prostatitis, 190
  testicular pain, 265 67, **266**
Rest in relieving
  angina, 1
  eyestrain, 91 92
  gout, 115
  migraine, 171
  muscle spasms, 181
  shinsplints, 219
  side stitches, 227
  sore throat, 234
  stubbed toe, 250
  testicular pain, 266
  toothache, 275
  wrist pain, 290
Rheumatoid arthritis, 7
RICE (rest, ice, compression, and eleva-
    tion) in relieving
  ankle pain, 5
  calf pain, 39–40
Rinses
  for cuts or scrapes, 69–70
  eye
    for corneal burns and abrasions,
      64–65
    for dislodging specks or dust, 88
  mouth
    for canker sores, 49
    for denture pain, 73
    for gum pain, 120–22, <u>120–21</u>
    over-the-counter, 121–22
    for pizza burn, 197–98
    for tongue pain, 270
    for toothache, 275
  saltwater, 73, 270, 275
  throat, 237

Rosemary, foot baths and, 115
Rotator cuff tendinitis, **38**
Rubbing alcohol, swimmer's ear and, 81
Running
  in swimming pool, 221
  tips for, <u>220</u>
Ruta graveolens, tennis elbow and, 263

S

Salt
  breast pain and, 25
  deficiency, 179–80, **228**
  kidney stones and, 159
Salves. *See* Ointments
Scabs, protection of, 71
Sciatica, **210–14**, <u>212</u>
Scrapes and cuts, **69–71**, <u>70</u>, **71**
Scrotal suspensory device, 266
Sedatives, neck pain and, 189
Sex positions, intercourse pain and, 153,
      192
Shaving, 204–5
Shield, bunion, 30–31
Shingles, **215–18**, <u>216</u>, **218**
Shinsplints, **219–22**, <u>220</u>, **222**
Shoes
  arch supports for, 32, 42
  blisters and, 21–22
  bunions and, 31
  calf pain and, 41–42
  corns and, 67–68
  foot pain and, 104
  good-fitting, 67, <u>102</u>, <u>135</u>, 149, <u>220</u>
  gout and, 116
  heel cushion in, 137
  heel pain and, 134, <u>135</u>
  heel-raiser for, 137
  ingrown toenail and, 148–49
  inner soles for, 42, 104, 162, 221
  stubbed toe and, 250
  varicose veins and, 284
Shoulder pain, **223–26**, **224**
Shoulder rolls exercise, 189
Shoulder shrugs exercise, 208
Side stitches, **227–29**, **228**

Boldfaced page references indicate main discussion of topic and "When to See the Doctor" boxes. <u>Underscored</u> page references indicate boxed text.

Silver. *See* Colloidal silver in relieving
Simethicone in antigas medications, 110
Sinus infection, <u>274</u>
Sinus pain, **230–33**, <u>231</u>, **232**
Sitting position
   back pain and, 13
   knee pain and, 163
   neck pain and, 186–87
   repetitive strain injury and, 207
   sciatica and, 211, 213–14
Skin care, 19
Skin problems. *See also* Blisters
   bedsores, 17–18, **18**
   burns, 33–35, **34**
   chafing, 54–56, **55**
   cuts and scrapes, 69–71, <u>70</u>, **71**
   psoriasis, **204**
   razor burn, 203–5, **204**
   shingles, 215–18, <u>216</u>, **218**
   splinters, 239–41, **240**
   sunburn, 251–54, **252**, <u>254</u>
   windburn, 286–88, **287**
Sleep
   migraine and, 171
   neck pain and, 188–89
   sinus pain and, 232
Smoking
   breast pain and, 26
   canker sores and, 49
   carpal tunnel syndrome and, 53
   coronary arteries and, 2
   fractures and, <u>142</u>
   gum pain and, 122
   irritable bowel syndrome and, 156
   pizza burn and, 198
   sinus pain and, 233
   sore throat and, 238
   temporomandibular disorder and, 257
   tongue pain and, 269
   ulcers and, 280
Snacks, hangover and, 125
Soaks. *See* Baths
Soaps
   chafing and, 55
   sunburn and, 252–53

Sodium. *See* Salt
Sodium bicarbonate. *See* Baking soda
     paste in relieving
Soles, inner shoe, 42, 104, 162, 221
Sorbitol
   gas pain and, 109
   in lozenges, throat, 74
Sore throat, **234–38**, <u>235</u>, **236**
Spasms, muscle, **181–84**, **182**
Spenco Second Skin, 34–35, 55
SPF, 62, 253, 288
Splinter forceps, 240
Splinters, **239–41**, **240**
Splints
   for bunions, 32
   wrist, **52**, 52–53, 291
Sports drinks, 123–24, 179
Sprain, ankle, **5**
Steam in relieving
   sinus pain, 231
   sore throat, 235–36
Steroids in relieving
   carpal tunnel syndrome, **42**
   cold sores, 62
Stockings, support, 284
Stomach acid, 132
Stomach pain, **242–47**, **244**
"Stone belt," 159
Stool, blood in, **109**
Stool softeners, 99, 139
Stress
   arthritis and, 9
   breast pain and, 26
   stomach pain and, 246
Stretching exercises, 144–45, <u>178</u>, 225
Stubbed toe, **248–50**, **249**
Sty, 89–90
Subungual hematoma, <u>147</u>
Sugar. *See also* Sorbitol
   menstrual pain and, 167
   raffinose, 110
   toothache and, 275
   ulcers and, 281
Sumatriptan (Rx), <u>173</u>
Sunburn, **251–54**, **252**, <u>254</u>

Boldfaced page references indicate main discussion of topic and "When to See the Doctor" boxes. <u>Underscored</u> page references indicate boxed text.

Sunglasses, corneal burns and abrasions
and, 63–64
Sun protection factor (SPF), 62, 253,
288
Sunscreen in preventing
cold sores, 62
sunburn, 253
windburn, 288
Supplements
DL phenylalanine, 168
fiber, 155
garlic, 79
lactase, 155
lysine, 61
vitamin C, 18, 62
zinc, 18, 50
Support groups for cancer pain, 44
Supports
arch, 32, 42
bra, 25–26
elbow, 263
knee, 162
neck, **188**
wrist, 291
Surgery
pain after, 199–202, **200**
in relieving
bunions, 32
carpal tunnel syndrome, **42**
corns, **68**
diverticulitis, 75
endometriosis, 86
Sweets. *See* Sugar
Swimmer's ear, 78–79, 81
Swimming, back pain and, 15

T

Tagamet HB, 245–46
Tai chi, back pain and, 16
Tanning, avoiding, 254
Tea
fennel, gas pain and, 109
with honey, sore throat and,
236–37
Tegretol (Rx), 196

Telephone receiver, holding
neck pain from, 187
repetitive strain injury from, 207
temporomandibular disorder from,
258
Temporomandibular disorder (TMD), **73**,
78, 95, **255–60**, 257, **259**, 274
Tendinitis, **38**, 291
Tendon, ruptured, 39
Tennis elbow, **261–64**, **262**, **263**
Tension headache, 126
Testicular pain, **265–67**, **266**
Tetanus shot, **71**
Thiamin deficiency, 259
Tic douloureux, 95
Tiger Balm, arthritis and, 9
TMD, **73**, 78, 95, **255–60**, 257, **259**,
274
Tobacco. *See* Smoking
Tongue pain, **268–72**, **269**, 270–71
Tooth, cracked, 273
Toothache, **273–77**, 274, **277**
Torsion, **266**
Transitions for Health, 86, 169
Tricyclic antidepressants, 196, 216
Trigeminal neuralgia, 95, 97
Tucks medicated pads, 139
Tweezers, splinters and,
239
Tylenol, 280
Tyramine, migraine and, 172, 173

U

Ulcers
gum, **118**, 121
mouth, **269**, 272
stomach, 278–81, **279**
Ulnar nerve, 291
Ultraviolet (UV) rays, protection from, 64,
251, 253, 254
Urea in hand cream, 29
Urethra, 152, 190
Uric acid production, 114–16
UV rays, protection from, 64, 251, 253,
254

Boldfaced page references indicate main discussion of topic and "When to See the Doctor" boxes. Underscored page references indicate boxed text.

V

Vaginal dryness, 151
Varicose veins, **282–85, 283**
Viadent mouthwash, gum pain and, 122
Vinegar in relieving
  chemical burn, 35
  swimmer's ear, 81
Visual distortions, 170
Visualization exercise, 45
Vitamin B$_6$
  breast pain and, 24–25
  carpal tunnel syndrome and, 53
  deficiency, 259
Vitamin C
  antioxidants in, 113
  bedsores and, 18
  burns and, 35
  cold sores and, 62
  deficiency of, 107
  genital herpes and, 113
  gout and, 116
  gum pain and, 122
  hangover and, 125
  muscle cramps and, 180
  overload, 125, 180, 259
  supplements, 18, 62
  temporomandibular disorder and, 259
Vitamin D, fracture prevention and, 142
Vitamin E
  breast pain and, 23–24
  vaginal dryness and, 151–52
Vitamins. *See specific types*
Vomiting, 245

W

Walking
  as back exercise, 15
  circulation and, 44
  metabolism of medications and, 44
  varicose veins and, 283
  in water, 144
Warm compress in relieving
  bursitis, 37
  ear pain, 79
  sty, 89

Water intake. *See* Fluid intake
Wax, orthodontic, toothache and, 276
Whiplash, 185, **188**
Windburn, **286–88, 287**
Wraps
  for cuts and scrapes, 69
  for muscle spasms, 183
  for phantom limb, 194
  for shingles, 218
Wrinkles, sunburn and, 251
Wrist pain, **289–92, 291**

X

Xylocaine Viscous (Rx), 271

Y

Yam-derived progesterone creams, 86,
  169
Yarrow, menstrual pain and, 168–69
Yawning, temporomandibular disorder
  and, 258
Yeast infections, 271
Yoga in relieving
  arthritis, 8
  back pain, 18
  hip pain, 145
  sciatica, 212–13

Z

Zilactin-B, cold sores and, 61
Zilactin in relieving
  canker sores, 50
  gum pain, 121
  pizza burn, 198
Zinc
  antioxidants in, 113
  bedsores and, 18
  burns and, 35
  canker sores and, 50
  genital herpes and, 113
  supplements, 18, 50
Zinc sulfate ointment, cold sores and, 61
Zostrix, 216
Zovirax (Rx), 111, 216

Boldfaced page references indicate main discussion of topic and "When to See the Doctor" boxes. Underscored page references indicate boxed text.